TH

Brenda Kidman has been a freelance writer and broadcaster since the BBC published her first book *A Handful of Tears* in 1974. She has written articles and stories for national publications and has been a regular contributor to 'Woman's Hour' and BBC Radio 4 with over 200 features and documentaries.

In 1977 Brenda had breast cancer. This made her realise the need for programmes which would deal frankly with this much-feared topic. Researching for her two Radio 4 documentaries, 'One Last Look at the Garden' and 'The Gentle Path', involved Brenda in a fascinating four-year study of so-called 'alternative' cancer therapies which convinced her that there was much more to the successful management of cancer than is at present offered by the medical establishment.

Brenda Kidman also made the award-winning radio documentary 'Where's the Key?' which is now a BBC/TV drama documentary. She is divorced with two sons and one grandson and lives in the wilds of Nottinghamshire.

ALEC FORBES MA, DM (Oxford), FRCP (London)

During 28 years as a Consultant Physician in Plymouth Hospital Alec Forbes became increasingly aware of the psychological and nutritional causes of disease, as well as the old and new approaches to health care. In 1977 he became a healer member of the National Federation of Spiritual Healers. Two years later the World Health Organisation appointed him advisor to its Traditional Medicine Programme. He left the NHS in 1980 to develop a working example of a new medical model for wholistic health care.

Part of the royalties from *A Gentle Way with Cancer* are being given to the Bristol Cancer Help Centre.

There is nothing so powerful
As an idea which has reached its time.

John Donne

Brenda Kidman

A Gentle Way with Cancer

What Every Cancer Patient
Should Know About the
Therapies which Can Influence
the Fight for Recovery

CENTURY PUBLISHING

LONDON

Copyright © Brenda Kidman 1983, 1985

First published in Great Britain in 1983
by Century Publishing Co. Ltd

Reprinted 1983 (twice)

New edition published in Great Britain in 1985
by Century Publishing Co. Ltd,
Portland House,
12-13 Greek Street, London W1V 5LE

ISBN 0 7126 0159 7

Photoset in North Wales by
Derek Doyle & Associates, Mold, Clwyd
Printed by The Guernsey Press Ltd,
Guernsey, Channel Islands

CONTENTS

Dedicated to cancer patients everywhere
who have been 'patient' long enough

AUTHOR'S NOTE

It's now seven years since I had cancer and conventional treatments for it. My introduction to the fascinating field of non-toxic cancer therapies came shortly afterwards when I was researching for a BBC radio documentary called 'The Gentle Path'.

It would be foolish to pretend that at first the gentle therapy measures for cancer control didn't fill me with confusion. They were, after all, a complete contradiction to my customary approach to health. Brought up in an era of state medicine, I was used to relying on my doctor to provide the remedies whenever I became ill. Then suddenly I was reading about measures which not only approached the dreaded illness of cancer with what seemed ridiculously simple methods, but also expected the patient to become a responsible participant in the fight for recovery.

Gradually, as I continued to research the subject of non-toxic therapies, a fundamental truth emerged. All gentle therapies do is to naturally create the internal conditions which stimulate the body's incredible ability to heal itself. This was an exciting revelation and one which has since given me an entirely new outlook on life and living. The logic behind the gentle cancer control therapies makes such good sense.

Many people I've talked to for this book have restored themselves to health by using both gentle methods and orthodox cancer treatments, allowing one approach to complement the other. In this way the patient has been able to have the best possible chance of getting well again. But there is another impressive attribute to gentle cancer therapies. The same measures which help the sick person combat disease can also be used to safeguard health once the principles involved are properly understood.

Of course cancer patients are all individuals. No two cases can be the same or treated in the same way. Adapting basic principles to suit individual needs means that the therapies described in this book do not comprise a 'do-it-yourself-anti-cancer-kit'. What they do provide is an insight into this illness called cancer and practical ways to combat disease and maintain health.

When Prince Charles addressed the British Medical Association on the occasion of their 150th Anniversary, he reminded them that: '... through the centuries healing has been practised by folk-healers who are guided by traditional wisdom that sees illness as a disorder of the whole person ... I would suggest that the whole imposing edifice of modern medicine, for all its breathtaking successes is ... slightly off balance ... The health of human beings is so often determined by their behaviour, their food and the nature of their environment ...'

These sentiments could herald a new age for cancer control if cancer patients choose gentle therapies and members of the medical profession adapt their expertise to incorporate them.

It is my fond hope that this book will provide readers with a stepping-stone to the gentle pathways to health and healing.

Brenda Kidman

FOREWORD

This book fills a pressing need to inform the public, the medical profession and the government about the existence of other valuable ways to treat cancer. This is not to imply that orthodox treatments should be abandoned. These will probably be needed for some time to come. In the meanwhile, it should be more widely realised that the fields of dietary and psychological change have much to offer in the control of this disease.

At present most of the money available for cancer research is directed at the investigation of scientific remedies. That is why for a long time now most research projects have concentrated on the biochemistry of immunity, virology and genetic transmission. As a consequence, very little of practical use in the successful long-term treatment of cancer has ever emerged. It is my belief that not until cancer research is viewed in much broader terms will any progress be made in the management of this distressing illness. I am also convinced that only when therapy measures are directed at correcting the spiritual, emotional and physical aspects of a degenerative disorder like cancer will the outlook for the control and prevention of this disease begin to show signs of improvement. Treating the symptoms is not enough.

I realise that it is easy to criticise the current medical model and its approach to the treatment of cancer. Unfortunately few doctors nowadays have the time to become involved in lengthy discussion with a patient to uncover the reasons for serious disease, let alone supply the psychological motivation which is a very necessary component for recovery.

This is why it is important that the general public become better informed about the nature of cancer and the deeper meanings of this illness. Only then can the wise patient begin to take some responsibility for actively helping the physician orchestrate the programme for recovery.

In the course of my work as a consultant physician over the last thirty years, I have repeatedly found that the patient prepared to make positive adjustments in his or her way of life has an improved chance of recovery compared with the patient content to drift passively along taking little or no interest in the prescribed treatments. Of course, struggling with a demanding disease like cancer requires hope and faith. Certainly nobody should live without hope for although this alone does not guarantee miracles, sustaining a positive attitude stimulates the body's natural self-healing abilities. Maintaining the patient's faith in the remarkable recuperative powers of the human body is also a vital ingredient in the recipe for recovery.

The total person approach for cancer control which we offer on an outpatient basis at the Bristol cancer Help Centre can, with modifications, also be applied to the treatment of all chronic illnesses. Our methods aim to establish within each individual patient the physical and mental conditions which first make it possible for the immune system to combat disease and then to regenerate 'ease'.

Since the Bristol centre opened in 1981, a steady stream of patients has been able to benefit from these largely self-help methods. This has encouraged us to find ways to expand the work of our charitable trust. Donations amounting to £100,000 enabled us to purchase larger premises which in 1983 were converted into a residential clinic staffed by qualified therapists and experienced volunteers. This places us in a strong position to demonstrate the tremendous value of the non-toxic programme for cancer control as outlined in Chapters 6, 7 and 8 of this book.

I believe that *A Gentle Way with cancer* provides a valuable introduction to comparatively simple therapies which cancer patients can use to help themselves get well again. That is why I do not hesitate to give this book my professional blessing.

Alec Forbes, Bristol, January 1983

1 DAVID'S STORY

The mother of a young university student wrote this when first she learned that her son had an inoperable brain tumour:

> The power of the word CANCER is overwhelming. It drives out the light and darkness pervades every waking moment. Fear grips with intensity, setting in motion negative reactions. You can no longer think rational thoughts or act with common sense. Suddenly you are helplessly caught up in the 'cancer machine' and brought face to face with death.
>
> Doctors give evasive answers. There's pity in their eyes but they cannot meet the pleading for hope in yours.
>
> 'David has perhaps another year at most,' they told me. 'If the radiotherapy works.'

In 1977 David Sutcliffe went up to Exeter University to study law. He soon got used to his fellow students' teasing suggestion that what he was really studying was not law but 'snore'. However much he fought against it, each day, and at totally inappropriate moments, David briefly fell asleep.

Not surprisingly at the end of his first year he failed his examinations. When he should have been studying, David was sleeping.

Suspecting that he might have some left-over symptoms from a bout of glandular fever which he'd suffered shortly after leaving home to go to college, on three occasions David went to his GP for a check-up. Each time he was given a clean bill of health.

'I tried to explain that I was finding it hard to concentrate on my work and kept falling asleep, but my doctor was always very busy. I got the impression he thought I was a bit of a hypochondriac. In fact I began to think so too.'

Although David sat his exams again, once more he failed them and had to leave university. This didn't upset him too much. Although he'd done well at school and got several A-levels, he wasn't particularly interested in an academic life. His real love was for the countryside and soon after leaving university he went to work on a farm in Somerset.

Doing a job he thoroughly enjoyed, for a while David felt fit and wide-awake. Then one day, as he was peering over his shoulder to back a tractor into an outbuilding, he realised that instead of seeing only one doorway, he could see two.

During the next two years, David suffered frequent headaches and bouts of double vision; but he still went ahead and enrolled at agricultural college at Cirencester, planning to begin his studies in Autumn 1980. But Sue Sutcliffe was worried about her son's health. Although she couldn't exactly put her finger on it, she thought David looked 'strange'.

A family friend, who was a doctor in Yeovil, was consulted. David fell asleep during his blood tests and ECG – a test of the electrical currents produced by his brain. The verdict was the same as before. There was nothing wrong with him. It was gently suggested that perhaps he tended to be over-anxious.

'Go away and have fun. Stop worrying about yourself,' was the professional advice.

Reassured that his symptoms were insignificant, David went abroad to get further farming experience in Australia and New Zealand, and while working there he did feel reasonably well.

'Must have been all those lamb chops for breakfast,' he said. Then, when the time came to return home, David decided to visit Bangkok. Within days he was running a high fever. Cabling his family in Somerset, he booked a seat on the next flight to Heathrow, where he was met by his two brothers. He looked so ill they hardly recognised him.

This time David's GP got him into Yeovil hospital for tests and para-typhoid was diagnosed.

While David was in hospital being treated for this, Sue mentioned to the doctor the muscle deterioration she'd noticed on one side of David's face.

'The doctor looked at me pityingly,' she remembered. 'He said that everyone has asymmetrical features.'

At the beginning of the Autumn term, David returned to college. As before he had to face the good-natured taunts of his fellow students; only this time they teased him about his appearance. David was 22 but resembled a middle-aged man of 40.

'One side of my face had sort of sagged. I found it difficult to speak clearly and I walked with a distinct lurch.' And once again he was seriously troubled by double vision.

Thinking that he probably needed a change of spectacles, David made an appointment to see an optician in Sherborne. The optician referred him to an eye specialist and two months later, in November 1980 and nearly three years after he had first suspected he was unwell, David received his first X-rays.

A few days afterwards, David got a 'phone call at the cottage he shared with fellow agricultural students. It was his mother.

'Now don't panic, but I've got the results of your X-rays,' she said, her voice struggling to remain steady. 'Apparently there's some kind of lump in your brain. They want to do some more tests.'

Far from being shocked by this news, David vividly remembers his sense of relief. Here at last was proof that he hadn't been imagining his strange symptoms. 'Now they'll do something about them,' he thought.

Events moved quickly. Within a week of Sue's 'phone call, David was at the Neurological Department of the Frenchay Hospital in Bristol having a brain scan. Soon afterwards he was admitted to the ward for more extensive tests.

'They had to do a special set of X-rays,' he explained. 'They pushed a catheter into my brain and injected dies while they flashed off pictures. I was told to lie still but it felt like a red-hot poker in my head. I know I screamed. I couldn't help it.'

After David had spent another three days flat on his back in hospital, his consultant finally gave him the diagnosis.

'He sat on my bed, fiddling with his pen, and said: "There's an abnormal growth in your brain-stem. It's called an astrocytoma".'

This is David's recollection of what was said although the same surgeon told his mother that her son's tumour was inoperable and invariably proved fatal.

A few days after Christmas 1980, Sue Sutcliffe took David and the rest of the family to a Christian healing service at Sherborne. She felt this was an important preparation for the deep X-ray treatment which the Bristol consultant had arranged. Although astrocytomas seldom responded to radiotherapy, there was a remote possibility that this treatment would retard the growth.

Early in 1981, trying to conceal her misgivings, Sue Sutcliffe drove her son the 45-mile journey from their home to the Frenchay Hospital in Bristol for David's first session of X-rays. David recalled this with horror.

On the third day he felt as though his head was going to explode and begged for an end to the treatment. Steroids provided some relief from the headaches but not from the nausea.

When he'd first gone for the treatment, David was in reasonably good physical shape. As the force of the X-rays began to take effect, he rapidly lost weight, felt perpetually cold and became extremely depressed. As his mother recalled, it was a desperate time for all the family.

'We understood so little about cancer. It was always something which happened to other people not to you. David's cancer was a terrible shock. Everyone in our family relied on David. He was the quiet, dependable one and although my five children have all been close to me, David was always a little bit special. Whenever I felt low, he was the one to provide a shoulder to lean on. Faced with his imminent death, we felt helpless and extremely frightened.

'Then one day a wise friend said to me: "You know you've got to give David up." The truth of this was hard to accept but I knew what she meant. If I truly loved David I shouldn't complicate his last months by refusing to face up to the fact that he was going to die. And I must somehow find the strength to help him and the other children to face this terrible crisis.

'It's not generally known that the Church of England offers confession. Since my marriage had broken up, I'd harboured a lot of resentment and hurt for many years. At first, confession didn't seem to make any difference. Then, a few weeks afterwards, I suddenly realised the bitterness had gone. In its place was a wonderful sense of inner strength which I knew would be a powerful source to draw upon in the months to come.

'I no longer anticipated the loss of David with such abject fear. I knew I could give him up.'

At this point David's story ceased to be one of despair and became instead one of hope. It was as if by freely relinquishing that which she treasured most, his mother had cleared the way for other possibilities.

In late January 1981, during the course of casual conversation, a friend asked Sue Sutcliffe if she'd heard about the newly opened Cancer Help Centre in Bristol.

Beginnings

Although healing was once an integral part of the Christian ministry, nowadays healing services are not a regular feature of church life. By and large, healing has become the responsibility of doctors not priests. But the Rev. Christopher Pilkington and his wife Pat always considered that healing was an important part of their pastoral duties.

'When we were bringing up our children,' Pat Pilkington recalled, 'if they were ill it was healing first and, if necessary, our doctor afterwards.'

In 1968 the Pilkingtons left their parish at Bromsgrove, Worcestershire, and moved to the parish of St Stephen's in Bristol. In addition to normal services, once every week Pat and her husband held meetings in the church to offer sick parishioners meditation and healing. But as the church was a popular tourist attraction, there were frequent interruptions.

The Pilkingtons longed for somewhere private to develop this side of their work and when, in 1975, Chris's father died and left them a substantial legacy, they bought a Victorian brownstone house at Downfield Road on the outskirts of Bristol and set up a small family charity called The Guy Pilkington Foundation. The house became both a healing centre and also somewhere for people to learn yoga and other forms of meditation and natural health methods.

'We felt we were fulfilling a need,' Pat Pilkington said. 'But we had no idea where this work would lead until one of our most staunch supporters suddenly became very ill with cancer.'

Penny Brohn, a qualified acupuncturist, had helped at Downfield Road since the centre had first opened. Then in one terrible year she lost both her parents. Within months she developed a particularly malignant type of breast cancer. Penny was then 36 and happily married with three young children at school.

Hospital consultants told her that a mastectomy might extend her life but in any event the outlook was grim. Penny's experience of 'alternative' medicine had taught her that disease was always a physical manifestation of a seriously disordered immune system. This was confirmed when Penny found *Cancer Another Way* by the Australian psychiatrist Dr Ainslie Meares. This doctor had for many years regarded cancer as a 'disease of the mind'. If she was to survive her cancer Penny realised she'd have to find a form of treatment which would revive her own natural self-healing defences.

That was in 1979. The NHS annual outlay for medical care was nearly £8 billion but none of this went to fund the giving of advice on the dietary control of cancer.

After carefully reading all the material she could find on the subject of nutrition and cancer, Penny decided this was the path to recovery she was going to follow. Although it meant borrowing the money to pay for the treatment, Penny put herself in the care of Dr Joseph Issels, the Bavarian doctor who for many years – and despite fierce opposition – has treated cancer with a special diet programme.

On two separate occasions Pat Pilkington flew out to spend a week with Penny at the lakeside clinic.

'She was desperately ill and, as she couldn't speak the language, felt really cut off and lonely. But gradually she began to respond to treatment.'

Often Pat and Penny talked about the future.

'It was really to cheer her up,' Pat recalled. 'When we fantasised about one day having a clinic in the UK where patients could have the same marvellous treatment Penny was getting. We didn't believe this would ever happen.'

After the second visit to Germany, Pat flew back to Heathrow Airport and drove down the M4 to Bristol. Before going home, she dropped in at Downfield Road to collect the mail. As she sifted through the bills and circulars, she came across one handwritten envelope.

It was from an old clergyman friend in Shropshire who for many years had been a prominent member of the Healing Research Trust, which amongst its members had a scattering of qualified medical practitioners who were also healers in the traditional sense.

'I know you've got a small house you use for the purpose of healing,' wrote the clergyman. 'I wonder whether you could help a good friend of mine called Dr Alec Forbes who is in Plymouth? He is looking for somewhere to set up a clinic where he can give cancer patients a programme of natural remedies.'

After reading this letter through several times, Pat still couldn't believe it.

'I'd just spent the whole week with Penny talking about

how we could get something going and there was this letter! In terms of my Christian teaching, this was divine guidance and could not be ignored.'

Dr Alec

In the immediate post-war years when the nation's health care services were just entering an era of medical technology and drug remedies, any NHS doctor who referred patients to so-called 'alternative' practitioners risked being struck off the medical register.

After the war, as Dr Alec Forbes settled down to civilian practice, he quickly realised that the state medical care model which was evolving, was one which was good at repair and reconstruction but had a poor record of success with chronic, degenerative diseases such as arthritis, diabetes, heart trouble and bronchitis. And, of course, the most feared disease of all – cancer. Gradually he realised that the most important factors causing disease were psychological and nutritional. He also became more aware of the dangers of modern drug remedies.

'Many of the patients who came into hospital for help had been given medicines which were supposed to be for "the treatment" of their disease,' Dr Alec said. 'But what we were seeing was the devastating and sometimes irreversible side-effects of drug treatments aimed at suppressing symptoms rather than dealing with the underlying causes of these illnesses.'

With cancer especially, Dr Alec became increasingly certain that the symptoms of this disease were the end results of long-term diet deficiencies and an unhealthy lifestyle which eventually caused serious changes in body chemistry. He also observed that quite often there were deep emotional problems involved with this chronic disorder, and accordingly began to study the psychological aspects of cancer and apply them to the treatment of some of his cancer patients.

His hospital colleagues viewed this bizarre approach with thinly veiled scepticism. However, upon Dr Alec's insistence, it was agreed that he could set up a trial where psychotherapy and healing would be given to cancer patients who had failed to respond to orthodox treatments.

Pleased at this apparent success, Dr Alec waited for the arrival of his first patients. None came. Eventually he tackled the oncology specialists who admitted that they hadn't the heart to refer patients to his clinic because this meant admitting that there was nothing further they could do to halt the disease.

Disappointed but undeterred, Dr Alec persevered with his development of the kind of health care which focused attention on the total person who was sick, not merely the disease. As he studied the nutritional therapy measures which were being used successfully by reputable practitioners in various other countries, Dr Alec was able to use his knowledge to help his patients, achieving results which conventional methods had mostly failed to produce.

And as time passed, his dissatisfaction with the style of medicine expected of him as a NHS hospital consultant continued to grow.

'My wife wanted me to resign,' he said. 'But I decided to stay on and be a bit of grit in the machine. The widespread increase of chronic ailments which we were seeing every day in the hospital was not just confined to the elderly but was increasingly affecting people of all age groups. I felt my colleagues would eventually have to concede that until they started tackling causes, they were not going to make much headway against this high incidence of degenerative illnesses.'

But although his professional colleagues chose to treat symptoms not causes, this did not deter Dr Alec from extending his individual efforts to provide 'wholistic' treatment.

Reports from various parts of the world were steadily confirming that cancer especially was a deficiency disease with emotional overtones.

Gradually the missing fragments of the cancer jigsaw were falling into place, and as the picture emerged so did two fundamental truths.

The cause and the control of cancer were the opposite sides of the same coin. And the depressing results of orthodox cancer treatments would continue so long as these were directed at the symptoms of disease and not at the whole person who had become sick.

'The medical profession with its increasing number of specialities,' said Dr Alec, 'divides patients into their component parts as if they were flesh-and-blood machines! This entirely overlooks the emotional and spiritual complexities which govern someone's state of health.'

Persevering with his own concept of what good medical practice was about, Dr Alec helped to found a network of Natural Health Centres up and down the country and spent much of his spare time addressing public meetings. Always the message was loud and clear. People would have to learn how to take positive steps to keep healthy if they wished to safeguard themselves against degenerative ailments. Prevention had to be the key since conventional medical treatments could not do much to help once faulty nutrition and bad habits had allowed the establishment of disease.

Throughout his career as a consultant physician within the NHS service, Dr Alec retained his optimistic conviction that eventually orthodox medicine would join forces with the best of naturopathic skills. Until such time, he had to content himself with doing what he could to utilise these principles within the limitations of his NHS medical practice, but he always longed for the chance to be able to offer this kind of health care on a wider basis.

Then, in 1979, Alec Forbes received a letter from Pat Pilkington in Bristol asking him to lecture at Downfield Road. He accepted.

Much of what Pat and Penny and the rest of the audience heard that evening was similar to the treatment Penny had received under Dr Issels. If Dr Alec could be persuaded to work at Downfield Road, the Bavarian fantasy could become an English reality! There was just one big snag. The Guy Pilkington Foundation was in no position to pay staff salaries.

Upon hearing this, Dr Alec's response was short and to the point.

'I'll work for nothing,' he said.

By midsummer of that year Dr Alec had resigned his post as Senior Consultant Physician at Plymouth Hospital and moved with his wife to Bristol.

The Truth About Cancer

Cancer is not an illness which strikes like a bolt from the blue. It is the result of a slow weakening of the body's defence and self-healing mechanisms aggravated by diet deficiencies and a generally inadequate lifestyle.

People in perfect health occasionally have cancer cells in their bodies. Some immunologists believe we actually produce thousands of cancer cells daily. Amongst the billions of cells continuously dividing, replicating and dying off in order to maintain healthy growth of bone, blood and tissue, it is hardly surprising that sometimes cells become faulty. These 'rogue' cells which fail to function in a normal, healthy way are soon recognised and destroyed by healthy body defences before they can cause any harm. Only when the immune system has been continuously sabotaged over a long period, does it then become possible for 'rogue' cells to form tumours.

But even then, what happens at a physical level is not the whole story. The whole story is, of course, the story of the *whole person* who has become progressively sick.

Poor diet lays the foundation for 80 per cent of cancer cases. Westerners may have plenty to eat, but due to modern methods of food production and processing much of this lacks the essential nutrients the body needs if it is to maintain an efficient immune system. Emotional stresses also affect body chemistry, and then there are environmental carcinogens which aggravate the formation of cancer cells. Industrial and agricultural pollutants in the air, soil and sea are prime examples of these. Lastly, there are the 'emotional carcinogens' often unwittingly woven into the thought-patterns of certain individuals, thus creating a natural susceptibility to the illness called cancer.

Gentle therapy measures are designed to regenerate and support the body's incredible ability to heal itself on all levels of being – physical, emotional and spiritual. In essence, this is what the 'wholistic' approach to cancer control is all about.

Laying Foundations

During the spring and summer of 1980, under the guidance of Dr Alec, the Downfield Road centre developed a therapy programme which it could offer to cancer patients wanting to become actively involved in their own fight for recovery.

Whilst working as a hospital physician, Dr Alec had frequently noticed that the well-informed patient who properly understood the nature of his illness and the personal effort needed to get well again, invariably did better than someone content to be the passive recipient of treatment.

So from the beginning, the regime outlined at the Bristol centre was specifically designed to encourage both the cancer patient and close family members to work together on the therapies involved.

On an out-patient basis, patients attending the centre were helped to learn how each part of the programme contributed to the overall daily approach to 'wholistic' living. This entailed preparation of a special diet of raw vegetables, salads and cereals, which vitamin supplements were necessary and how these interacted with additional supplements of enzymes and minerals. People learned how the relaxation and breathing exercises prepared them for the deeper state of meditation and the valuable mental imagery techniques which could have such an important bearing on recovery. And above all, patients would be offered counselling, healing and spiritual support.

The concept was brilliant. Under one roof were gathered a qualified physician and a staff of therapists able to attend to the mind, body and spirit of the sick person. But always Dr Alec and the Bristol Centre staff regarded wholistic treatments as valuable complementary measures, never alternatives for orthodox cancer care. In this way patients would be getting the best of both worlds in the fight for recovery. And the great advantage of the gentle therapies was that they were completely without harmful side-effects.

In October 1980 the Bristol Cancer Help Centre opened its doors to the public. Amongst the first people to cross the threshold were David Sutcliffe and his mother.

As Sue Sutcliffe immediately noticed, the moment she and David walked through the front door the welcome was one of warmth, love and understanding. Above all, everyone talked about cancer as if it was just like any other illness.

Step by step the Sutcliffes were introduced to the wholistic therapy programme and Sue realised that everything they were being told made tremendous good sense. If David was to have any chance of recovery, this was the route he had to follow.

Sue gave up her job in order to help David over the first weeks of the new daily routine. Dr Alec had fully explained how the diet and the vitamin therapy would cleanse David's system and what to expect when the body started to respond with the first of a series of 'healing crises'. At these times David would feel worse, not better, as his revived immune system destroyed the tumour and washed toxins into his bloodstream. Then frequent coffee enemas to stimulate his liver in its work of detoxification would relieve these symptoms.

The Sutcliffes had completely to reorganise their daily

lives in order to concentrate on the strict programme of juices and salads, the carefully spaced doses of laetrile injections (which their GP agreed to administer), and the other vitamins, enzymes and mineral supplements used in tumour destruction. Time had to be set aside for the coffee enemas and the three half-hour periods for the meditation exercises.

In the role of 'carer', Sue found it hard going in both practical and emotional terms. The bulk of each day was spent shopping for the diet and preparing it as well as running the household for the rest of the family. And she had to learn the best way to give David moral support during the early days when he felt it was all a waste of time. She had to judge when all he needed was gentle encouragement and the other times when he had to be bullied into sticking to the schedule.

Outside the home she encountered considerable resistance from relatives and friends.

'You do realise it's David's life you're playing with,' was one of the censorious remarks frequently levelled at her. Then there were neighbours who had once been regular visitors to the Sutcliffe house but who had stopped coming once they thought David was dying. In the village they sometimes crossed the street in order to avoid meeting Sue.

'It wasn't that these people didn't feel sympathetic,' Sue insisted. 'Only that they didn't know what to say for the best. They found it difficult to handle their own fear of cancer. Then it was up to us to put people at ease by showing that we didn't mind talking about it.'

Sue and David continued to go weekly to the Bristol Cancer Help Centre. And gradually David began to get stronger.

Shortly before Easter 1981, Sue bought a puppy to encourage David to take it for walks. Each time they went off together the walks grew longer. By the time the puppy was a handsome dog, David was feeling well again.

In June 1982 David Sutcliffe returned to his consultant for tests. The tumour on his brain had regressed and was no longer causing any symptoms.

'Being able to work together to help David through his illness has been a learning experience,' said Sue Sutcliffe. 'When David lost all his hair – when we spent so much time at the kitchen sink scrubbing carrots and cleaning the juicing machine, we had to see the funny side. I'm sure we are a wiser, stronger and more united family as a result.

'As for the people at the Centre, I owe them a debt of gratitude I'll never be able to repay ...'

Today Sue Sutcliffe is one of the therapists at the new Bristol Centre. Her own family experience makes her emminently qualified to counsel others going through a similar crisis. As for David, he now looks as fit as he feels.

A Special Kind of Caring

My first encounter with the Bristol Cancer Help Centre was in November 1980 when I went there to do some research for a radio documentary on new approaches for cancer. I remember walking in to the Downfield Road house and hearing the cheerful buzz of conversation coming from the lounge, the sound of food mixers whizzing in the kitchen.

No white coats, no aseptic corridors with labelled doors, no indifferent voices. Instead the atmosphere was one of sensible optimism. Here was real concern for individual needs combined with practical help often provided by therapists who had themselves started as patients.

Later that day, as I sat in the train staring out at the Gloucestershire countryside, my thoughts returned to the November of exactly three years before when I first discovered that I had cancer.

2   THE CONVENTIONAL THERAPY SCENE

One February night in 1977 I found a scarcely detectable lump on the outer side of my left breast. I was having a bath at the time. Despite the hot, steamy atmosphere I shivered. I was well aware of the possible implications of what I'd discovered.

That night was a restless one, disturbing dreams alternating with long periods of wakefulness when my fingers repeatedly explored that unfamiliar body contour in the remote hope that I'd imagined it. The last thing I wanted just then was a serious health problem.

I was 47 and just getting over the death of my mother and the difficult year which preceded it when she had suffered from an acute form of senile dementia. My attempts to look after her prevented me working as a radio journalist. Because his grandmother's long illness had caused as much disruption to my young son's life as it had to mine, it was essential to get our domestic and financial affairs back on an even keel.

So by daybreak I'd made up my mind. I would have to ignore that wretched little lump.

In retrospect, it is astonishing how little I knew about my predicament. I didn't even realise that swellings which appear in the breast aren't always malignant. Just before menstruation some women's breasts tend to feel lumpy but once menstruation begins, these lumps disappear.

Then again, more persistent swellings often turn out to be easily treated cysts called adenomas.

Nobody in my immediate family had ever suffered from breast cancer, otherwise I daresay I'd have been better informed about the subject. All I knew at the time was that successful treatment was supposed to depend on getting it sooner rather than later. I have since discovered that this 'early warning' propaganda doesn't help much when you understand the rate at which cancer tumours grow.

> Calculations show that a breast tumour begins between six and four years before it presents any symptoms. By the time the 'lump' is able to be felt it has already grown through the 30th doubling of its cells. Cancer tumours rarely grow beyond a 40th doubling which means that at present treatment is seldom started until the last quarter of the evolution of the disease which is terribly late ... (*Conquering Cancer* by Lucien Israel.)

Cancer specialists would probably argue that treatment at the 30th doubling is better than at the 31st. Once again there is contradictory evidence.

The mortality rate for breast cancer hasn't changed for the last 70 years and a third of women who get it don't survive more than five years after the initial diagnosis when given conventional treatments.

The claim that early detection improves survival chances is even less convincing when one reads in the *British Medical Journal* (July 1980) that, 'it seems likely that dissemination [spread] of disease beyond the breast may occur before the appearance of the first symptom, let alone initial diagnosis.'

Government sponsored campaigns offering routine tests to identify early symptoms of breast and cervical cancer have never publicised these discouraging facts about the growth and spread of tumours. These campaigns have been devised to reassure the public; but there are those who believe that the screening programmes cause more trouble than they prevent, certainly at an emotional level.

Whether it is for a Pap smear for cervical cancer or mammography for breast cancer, those who come forward for examination are bound to feel anxious.

Imagine the experience of a woman whose test indicates a pre-cancerous condition. She is asked to return in six months' time for another examination but told 'not to worry about it'. Six months is a long time to live with the possibility that you may have cancer even if, as frequently happens, the second test doesn't confirm the first.

Very little is known about the early development of

cancer. Skin blemishes like moles and warts are benign tumours and everyone knows how warts come and go. So it is not inconceivable that a pre-cancerous condition might appear and disappear according to the individual's state of health, bearing in mind that all of us have 'cancer cells' in the body from time to time and these are effectively eliminated by the healthy immune system.

Moreover, some women are known to have a cancerous condition of the cervix which never produces any troublesome symptoms. So the value of 'early warning' screening programmes is questionable.

Potentially Dangerous Diagnostic Methods For Breast Cancer

MAMMOGRAPHY

This is an X-ray technique (introduced in 1960) which builds up a series of pictures of internal tissue from several angles. In the USA it has been widely criticised as a routine procedure to detect possible malignancy because it exposes women to the risk of cumulative X-ray damage.

THERMOGRAPHY

This is a safer diagnostic procedure than mammography. The technique is based on the fact that malignant growths radiate more heat than healthy tissue. So thermography of a woman's breasts builds up an infra-red picture. Cancerous cells show up as dark spots.

Compared with mammography this heat technique was not found to be a reliable method of early detection in the States when cross-checked by other diagnostic methods. Out of 160 women pronounced clear by thermograms 97 were subsequently found to have detectable growths.

ULTRASONOGRAPHY

This is a safe and simple diagnostic method increasingly used in all the larger hospitals. A medical development of a wartime detector device based on SONAR, the ultrasonograph 'pencil' is moved over the patient's body, bouncing sound frequencies off internal organs which are computorised to present a screened image for the diagnostician.

TOTAL BODY SCANNERS

In many cases, a 'scan' is a routine precautionary procedure within a year of surgery or other cancer treatments. The patient reports to the hospital department a few hours prior to the scan. An injection of radioactive material is given. The content of this varies according to whether it is soft body tissue or bone which is to be examined. Radio-isotopes become evenly distributed throughout healthy tissue but cannot permeate malignant cells.

The patient lies on a bed under the scanner which picks up signals from the radio-isotopes and transmits these onto a monitor screen. As the picture builds up the diagnostician is able to identify and locate the presence of tumours which show up as isolated dark areas amongst the pinpoints of brightness emitted by the radio-isotopes.

NUCLEAR MAGNETIC RESONANCE

This is a comparatively new type of diagnostic scanner which can examine the brain and other parts of the body without the use of radioactive materials and in three-dimensional 'pictures'. It works by placing the patient in a magnetic field and by emitting radio pulses which stimulate signals in the atoms of the body. Cancer cells emit radio frequency signals which differ from healthy cell emissions and these are picked up and displayed on a monitor screen.

At present NMR scanners cost in the region of half-a-million pounds each and only a few British hospitals are equipped with them.

But the same basic objections may be levelled at all these attempts to pinpoint early cases of cancer. Microscopic tumours probably come and go due to the efficiency of the body's natural defence system. The only positive benefit from an early warning device would be to alert the individual to the fact that it was time to start doing something positive about a lifestyle which was obviously undermining his or her health.

In *World Medicine* (1980) Professor Roger Cotton, who is head of the Diagnostic Oncology Department at Nottingham's City Hospital, describes an investigation which checked up on 100 women whose cervical smears were positive but for various reasons went untreated. He was able to show that amongst those who returned for a further examination several years afterwards, some revealed no sign of cancer whilst others showed that the 'cancer' was still there but had given them no trouble.

Again, the inference is that even when cancer tumours form in the body it is possible for the immune system to contain them in a harmless condition.

So my decision not to consult my GP immediately after I found that small lump in my breast was after all not so foolish.

In the year following its discovery I often completely forgot about my little lump. It was painless and did not get any larger. Then towards the end of 1977 I happened to be in my BBC producer's office when she was compiling a programme for 'Woman's Hour' about breast prosthesis. She had a sample one in a box and showed it to me. The pliable pink bag had an artificial nipple moulded onto it.

'Hope I never need one of these,' I said half jokingly. She gave me a quizzical look.

'What makes you say that?' she said.

'Well, I don't expect it's of any consequence, but I've had this pea-sized lump in my breast for nearly a year now. If it was anything serious it would have grown larger, wouldn't it?'

'You must be mad,' she retorted and proceded to give me the benefit of all the research she'd been doing for her programme.

'Be sensible and get your doctor to look at it,' she finally recommended. 'Then at least one way or the other you'll know what it is.'

A week later I presented myself at my doctor's evening surgery. I'd been registered with him for two years but this was our first meeting.

'I'm not ill,' I remember saying. 'In fact I feel extremely fit. It's just this stupid little bump I've had for a while now.'

After examining me his suggestion that I see a specialist was made so casually no alarm signals sounded in my head. All I felt was a mild sense of annoyance that I'd have to take time off work to keep the appointment. If I kept it. He must have read my thoughts.

'No need to lose any sleep over this little lump,' he assured me in his attractive Scottish accent. 'But I always send my ladies for an expert opinion so be sure to keep the appointment now.'

Which is how in late October of that year I found myself sitting in the crowded corridor which served as the outpatient waiting area in our local hospital.

When confronted by my 'lump' the consultant surgeon appeared no more impressed than my GP. He'd probably seen more mammalian protuberances than I'd had hot dinners!

'It's really very small,' he remarked but even as I started to apologise for wasting his time, said: 'But to be on the safe side we'll get you into hospital for a biopsy.'

He briefly explained that under a general anaesthetic the growth would be excised and sent for laboratory analysis. If benign I would be discharged the following day.

'And if it isn't?' I asked, my mouth suddenly dry.

'Then I'm afraid you'll lose your breast,' he replied, holding open the door to the corridor.

My oldest son was on leave from the Royal Navy so a week later he was able to drive me to the hospital. By then I was feeling extremely frightened although determined not to show it. In a health service renowned for long waiting lists, I'd been allocated a bed with a haste that could only mean one thing. I was considered in need of emergency treatment. Yet I didn't feel the slightest bit ill.

In the light of what I've learned since, I find it incredible that I never for a single moment paused to question what was happening. But then I'd been brought up to regard all doctors as authority figures. It never crossed my mind that I could make my own decisions about what should be done with my body!

On a bright, cold November morning I reported to the hospital ward. It was the modern open-fronted kind, six-bed sections fronting on to a wide corridor with floortiles polished to the consistency of glass. Mingled with the shivery smell of antiseptic was the more comforting aroma of boiled cabbage.

My bed was under a large metal-framed window with a bird's eye view of the high-rise city centre, an industrial curve of the river and, below, a public park where tides of brown leaves washed across skeletal rosebeds.

Behind the curtains surrounding my bed I transferred the contents of my overnight bag to the locker; toilet things, pens and notebook, a box of tissues, my purse and a Henry James novel.

Rather than give my sons the bother of laundering nighties, I'd decided to wear hospital issue. This turned out to be a voluminous flannelette affair with gaping neckline. Folding my outdoor clothes into a large polythene carrier, I put on the nightgown and climbed into bed. As the nurse swished the curtains back and disappeared with my clothes I felt I had lost the last links with individuality. Now I was a number in a bed.

Reaching for the paperback I tried to concentrate on the

Victorian world within. Between visits from the house-surgeon, the lab technician and various nurses, from the physiotherapist and the ward secretary, I read my book. Pricked by needles, baring my bosoms for young medical students, taken for X-rays and exhaustively questioned for a slowly fattening folder of paperwork, although my eyes moved across the lines of print and my finger turned the pages, I was unable to recall one single sentence.

Cheerfully processed along the medical conveyor belt, I felt like some kind of modern-day Pearl White chained to the tracks of an on-coming train! Except that I knew instinctively that there'd be no last minute rescue for me. I was about to pay dearly for my procrastination.

During the remainder of that day my one positive contribution to the entire proceedings was misconstrued.

A young woman medical student wanted to write up my case history. This involved a meticulous résumé of all my health problems. As she scribbled away I suddenly remembered the Kidney Donor Card which I'd been carrying since I once made a radio programme with some youngsters on dialysis. Taking the card from my wallet I tried to hand it to her but she waved it aside.

'Don't be so morbid,' she exclaimed. 'We shan't need *that*!' This one attempt to take some responsibility for my own body, was rejected.

By the end of the day I was in the grip of gut-curdling fear. The following morning I'd be taken to the operating theatre. I'd already signed the 'consent form' which gave my surgeon permission to remove the growth in my breast for a 'frozen section'. This was a laboratory technique which produced a microscopic slice of tissue for examination. According to the result, either the wound in my breast would be sewn up or the breast removed. Until I recovered consciousness I wouldn't know which.

Towards evening of that first day in hospital, the preliminaries completed, I was left alone with my thoughts. If only there'd been someone qualified to sit down and discuss with me all the implications of my illness, at that

point I should have welcomed this attention. I wanted to
know exactly what was meant by 'losing a breast' but was
afraid to ask.

In my ignorance I supposed it would be sliced off to leave
a large expanse of raw flesh. If this happened, I wondered
how long it would take to convalesce and get back to work?
And if the breast was removed, did this mean that I'd been
cured of cancer?

Painful though the answers might be, I badly needed
someone to spell out exactly what the future held in store.

What I didn't realise when I signed the 'consent form'
was that I could have given my consent for the biopsy only
and been returned to the ward minus no more than the
offending lump. This would have given me an opportunity to
ask the questions I needed answers to and adjust to the idea
of an amputation supposing the lab report was positive.

Nor did I know at the time that there are excellent
reasons for separating the biopsy from more radical
procedures.

A frozen section is done at speed so an instant report can
be relayed to the surgeon in the operating theatre. Only
later is this report followed by an examination of a properly
stained section which takes days to complete. The second
test should confirm the first but what if the surgeon acts on
the first positive report and the second doesn't confirm it?
Unless surgery is a matter of emergency, a time lapse
between the biopsy and the next step is a sensible
precaution. Even laboratory technicians are not infallible.

Married women especially can make good use of this
two-stage procedure. This not only allows time for all those
questions which only gradually come to mind, but gives the
family an opportunity to rally round and provide moral
support at a time when a woman needs all she can get.

As the hands on the ward clock crawled round the face,
on that first night in hospital I fervently wished there was
someone to reassure me. It was a lonely experience, lying
there listening to the loud snoring which came from the
woman in the bed by the door, hearing occasional bursts of

half-stifled laughter from the nurses' post in the corridor or the far-off wail of an ambulance siren somewhere out in the city.

Next morning, whilst the other patients ate breakfast, I was given my pre-medication.

The hair was shaved from my armpits and pubic area, my head enveloped in a large paper mob-cap. A short white cotton gown which tied at the back and thick woollen socks completed the regulation attire.

At a time when my morale had hit rock bottom, these ugly garments obliterated the last traces of self-confidence. But even as I was wondering what piece of thoughtless bureaucracy forced someone facing major surgery to dress like a clown, orderlies arrived with the theatre trolley.

My return to consciousness was accompanied by angry resentment. Efficient but none too gentle hands were rolling me first one way and then another as the canvas trolley stretcher was dragged out from under my back. It felt as though someone had clamped a branch of holly under my left armpit and the rest of my body had been reduced to a helpless pulp. All I wanted was to sink back into oblivion, to escape the ripping pain which brought frantic wounded-animal sounds from my throat.

At last they gave me an injection and went away. As delicious waves of sleep softened the pain, I moved my right hand to my left shoulder. It found a flat gauze dressing and tubes. My breast had gone.

The day after the operation, the surgeon and his posse of students arrived at the foot of my bed.

'You were lucky,' he said with a note of reproval in his voice. 'It hadn't spread.' I didn't feel lucky. I felt wretched. As well as the pricking, stabbing pain in my armpit, there was the discomfort of two thick drainage tubes stitched into stab-wounds in my chest and connected to a pair of vacuum jars hanging on a rack beneath the bed. Until the tubes were removed five days after the operation, wherever I went the bottle rack went too. I shuffled about the ward like Dracula's milkman!

I suppose that I had expected to lose my breast. What I wasn't prepared for was the effect this amputation had on my left arm which had become swollen from shoulder to elbow and devoid of strength.

Two days after my mastectomy, when the nurse changed the dressing, I squinted down at my new chest. There was a line of stitches on a horizontal scar which extended from centre front to just behind my left armpit.

'Good for you!' the nurse congratulated. 'So often our mastectomy ladies are too upset to look.'

This I could understand. I was horrified to see that my remaining breast, deprived of its partner, resembled a commemorative monument erected on a disaster site! How could such an insignificant lump have caused such havoc? Nor was it any consolation to identify the remains of my left nipple in the scar. Along with that amputated breast had gone an essential part of my feminine sexuality.

The surgical removal of a woman's breast inflicts both physical and emotional wounds especially in a society where buxom breasts are an important attribute of female attractiveness.

But for me the unkindest cut of all was the end result of all this mutilation. I'd been transformed from an apparently fit woman into yet another cypher in the national cancer statistics.

There are more than 40,000 cases of breast cancer in the UK each year and whereas once it was mostly women over 60 who developed it, in the last decade much younger women have fallen victim to this disease.

A large proportion of the £37m spent annually on cancer research is on researching remedies for breast cancer, but despite this expenditure, treatment procedures have changed little since the beginning of the century, and some form of surgery is almost always indicated.

Varieties of Surgery for Breast Cancer

LUMPECTOMY

This is the least extensive operation for breast cancer. The tumour is removed with a little surrounding tissue and this hardly alters the contour of the breast. Since 1983 and the publicity given to the subject of breast cancer, lumpectomies have gained surgical respectability as a first line of surgical intervention.

WEDGE RESECTION

Surgery involving the removal of a wedge-shaped portion of the breast and possibly some of the lymph nodes in the armpit if infected, only leaves the breast slightly disfigured. However removal of lymph glands can cause long-term problems with the arm on the side of surgery.

SIMPLE MASTECTOMY

This amputates all the breast tissue. As many women can testify, a surgical legacy of exposed nerve endings can often be the cause of chronic pain and discomfort long afterwards.

MODIFIED RADICAL MASTECTOMY

With this the entire breast and any apparently abnormal lymph nodes in the armpit are removed.

RADICAL MASTECTOMY

This goes a stage further than modified radical mastectomy and removes all the lymph nodes in the armpit and the pectoral muscles. This is a very disfiguring procedure which is now rarely performed in this country.

SUBCUTANEOUS MASTECTOMY

This is the only new surgical procedure for breast cancer
introduced in the last 15 years. The internal breast tissue is
removed leaving the nipple and enough skin to enable a
silicone implant at a later date. This eventually restores a
permanent shape to the breast but is a controversial
procedure. Leaving any part of a cancerous breast, it is
argued, may also leave tumour cells which could start to
grow again. So this operation is only offered to a woman
when the consultant feels psychological benefits would
appear to outweigh medical risks. As for the ordinary NHS
mastectomy patient, a prosthesis which is a tolerable replica
of her remaining breast is supplied to fit into her brassière.

The need for cancer patients to want to blame someone or
something for their illness is a very natural reaction, even
when many suppositions have no basis in fact.

For instance, cancer is not contagious. Nor is it inherited,
although certainly the patient's faulty lifestyle may well be
conditioned by family habits which are passed from one
generation to another. Nor is cancer the result of an
accidental knock, although a serious accident which causes
stress could trigger off cancer in someone with a
predisposition to the disease.

Many people believe that surgery will make a cancer
spread. The truth is that most tumours shed stray
malignant cells into the bloodstream which may or may not
form 'secondary' growths depending upon the efficiency of
the individual's own natural body defence system. But it is
true that in some cases cancer patients die quickly after
surgery and this has prompted the speculation that exposing
the tumour to air may speed up its rate of growth. Enclosed
in the body, cancer cells which reproduce by the process of
sugar fermentation, will grow slowly over a long period. It
has been suggested that oxygen could accelerate tumour
growth and thus precipitate fatal conclusions.

But when a tumour is causing a vital obstruction there is no alternative for the patient but to submit to surgery.

Within a week of my operation I was able to spend most of each day in the ward dayroom. It was then that I discovered that while other patients chatted freely about their operations, once I mentioned the word cancer in connection with mine, there was an abrupt change of subject.

The medical staff also avoided using the taboo word. Instead they talked euphemistically of my 'nasty little lump', 'growth', or 'tumour' or merely referred to cancer, as my consultant had done, by saying 'it'.

This reluctance on the part of my fellow patients to discuss my illness made me feel isolated. I'd no idea I'd contracted a disease which carried with it a social stigma, especially in a liberated society where full-frontal attitudes to everything were supposed to have banished all inhibitions.

At first I was upset. I hadn't asked to join an élite group of unmentionables. Only when I started to consider the background to such ingrained behaviour did it become more understandable. And part of the blame is rooted in the way our National Health Services have created a state monopoly on health care.

Immunisation and vaccination for infectious diseases such as smallpox, malaria, cholera, typhoid, polio, diptheria and the other recurring epidemics which from time to time decimated the population, provided mass protection to the community.

Then came antibiotics to eliminate the potentially fatal threats of tuberculosis, pneumonia, meningitis, septicaemia and venereal disease.

By the 1950s 'instant' medication in the form of drug remedies was being freely prescribed. Allopathic practitioners seemed to have all our health problems neatly under control. Getting ill was no longer a traumatic event.

National Health Insurance took care of the costs, doctors took care of the diseases and a generation growing up in a climate of 'live now pay later' were happy to abdicate personal responsibility for their health care. We became a nation of humpty-dumpties confident that the medical profession would put us together again whenever we fell off the wall.

Today the complexities of treatments on offer are beyond the understanding of the average patient.

Electron microscopes enable scientists to unravel the innermost secrets of human creation, television spectaculars feature surgeons working with human hearts and life-support technology. No wonder the average citizen continues to dread cancer when it casts its long shadow over the dazzling exploits of our medical mechanics. Having put our trust in them, the realisation that no amount of technical expertise or financial investment has succeeded in conquering cancer, taints the whole subject with an aura of despair.

Charitable fund-raising agencies unwittingly compound this public unease. Using grim statistics (cancer kills 145,000 people in the UK each year) to encourage donations, cancer charities pour millions (nearly £40 million in 1983) into research projects recommended by orthodox cancer specialists, inevitably focused on perpetuating cancer machinery and drug treatments.

Such is the prestige of the medical profession, everybody is persuaded that one day the scientists will produce the magical cancer cure. Quick to seize a sensational headline, the media reinforce this impression whenever they publish a story about the latest 'medical breakthrough' on the cancer front. Hopeful hearts start beating – until the acid truth is revealed. The most notorious example of this, was interferon.

In 1980 a story in *Time* magazine hailed interferon as the 'Miracle Drug', a substance supposed to interfere and slow down the growth of malignant tumours. Tens of thousands of cancer sufferers beseiged cancer organisations for a chance to be given treatment, only to be told that interferon would not be available until it had been subjected to further investigation.

Using the publicity surrounding this report to its advantage, the American Cancer Society immediately launched a campaign to raise funds for interferon research. Hopeful people everywhere contributed more than 15 million dollars before, that same year, a cancer specialist in Glasgow published an article in the *British Medical Journal*, pointing out that the claims being made for interferon were grossly exaggerated.

Out of eighteen cancer patients treated with interferon, two had shown a brief improvement, but these also died once treatment was suspended. Only then did the public learn the brutal facts about the 'wonder drug'.

Had interferon proved beneficial, not only would dosage have had to be continued indefinitely, but there were serious side-effects attached to this treatment. And, to cap it all, it was revealed that in order to extract a fraction of an ounce of interferon required more than 100,000 pints of human blood!

Only last year another sensational cancer treatment was announced in a national paper: 'UK Surgeons Test "Anti-Cancer" Ray'. Whether this also proves irresponsible reporting remains to be seen. But is it any wonder that the belief that cancer is some kind of incurable juggernaut continues to sustain our worst fears and leaves us clinging to the possibility of a scientific solution to the exclusion of all else? As we shall see, the truth of the matter is far less frightening.

After nine days in hospital, I went home for Christmas. The bedroom mirror reflected the face of a weary octagenarian. My innermost thoughts were far worse. Without any idea of how long it would take to regain my strength, I was desperately afraid of what the future might hold.

Shortly before Christmas I reported to my surgeon for the first in the series of check-ups which would become a regular feature over the next five years as my progress, or lack of it, was officially charted. If, at the end of five years, I had a clean bill of health I would go down in the official cancer statistics as having survived. (One out of three women 'survive' mastectomy.)

That December, as I waited again in the local hospital corridor, I doubted I'd survive one year let alone five. And mixed with this pessimism was a sense of utter helplessness.

How could I fight a disease which had struck so suddenly and turned me from a healthy person into a physical wreck?

If I'd privately decided there was nothing I could do to help myself, my surgeon had definite plans for my immediate future. After he'd inspected my red-raw scar and pressed his fingers into my armpits, he suggested a course of radiotherapy to 'kill off any stray cancer cells still lurking in my chest'.

'But I thought you said I was lucky that it hadn't spread,' I protested, sensing a betrayal.

'I removed four invaded lymph glands from your axilla,' he informed me, ignoring the inference that he'd concealed the truth of my condition. But the question of just how frank a doctor should be with a cancer patient has always aroused a good deal of controversy.

To Tell or Not To Tell

Referred to by the medical profession as 'therapeutic deception', until the late 1950s the policy of most British doctors was to conceal the truth.

For a long time it was argued that because in most people the word cancer generated entirely negative reactions, informing the patient that he had this disease would cause him to turn his face to the wall and give up. However, this was obviously a policy which not only perpetuated negative attitudes but reflected on the doctor's professional image, since when a patient died and the cause of death was entered on the death certificate, the family's worst fears about the incurability of cancer were confirmed. Then again, the policy of 'not telling' helped to propagate the gospel of despair, because when a *recovered* cancer patient was later told of the true diagnosis, he tended to believe the doctor had made a mistake in the first place!

So this conspiracy of silence invariably meant that in the public mind cancer grew to be a disease synonymous with death.

A hospital survey done in Manchester in the early 1950s was a fair indication of this. Of those asked if they thought cancer was an incurable disease, 64 per cent believed this to be true.

Then, in 1959, the famous Christie Hospital in Manchester conducted another survey. Entitled 'Patient Reaction to Being Told of Their Diagnosis' this revealed that out of hundreds of interviews with patients to discover whether or not they wanted their doctors to tell them if they had cancer, it was shown that only 7 per cent positively resented the idea of being told. Furthermore, it also emerged that more women than men (one third more) expressed the need to be told the truth.

Twenty years on, thanks to the courage of patients prepared to talk openly about having cancer, and numerous radio and television documentaries as well as programmes which give people an opportunity to discuss this hitherto taboo subject, attitudes are changing. And doctors also are finding that by creating an honest relationship with their cancer patients, the well-informed patient tends to co-operate better with the treatments advised.

More importantly, a number of university hospital studies have, in the last decade, clearly shown that when an open approach is combined with counselling and psychotherapy, the patient's response to treatment is much improved.

The Radiotherapy hostel where I spent three weeks undergoing treatment was for patients who lived too far away to attend for daily treatment.

There were about 30 of us, men and women, collected together in what amounted to a cancer ghetto. The hostel resembled a boarding house. The food served in the ground-floor dining-room with check tablecloths was the pre-cooked, pre-heated and otherwise tasteless variety. Lots of greasy chips, frozen or tinned vegetables, bulk-baked meat pies and instant desserts appeared with remorseless regularity. Occasionally there was fresh fruit.

On the first floor of the hostel were two sitting-rooms, the smaller for the men, the larger one for us women. Identical armchairs were lined up against the walls. There was a scattering of wickerwork footrests and low tables, a colour television set in the bay window and little else.

Most of the bedrooms were up another flight of stairs. The gloomy dormitory on the ground floor was reserved for those too ill to climb stairs.

Although our continual presence offered a captive audience for health education, cancer counselling and physiotherapy, these were not provided. Between treatments the men smoked, filled out football coupons and played cards. The women knitted, gossiped and discussed *Coronation Street* – until it was time to switch the programme on.

Soon after breakfast we walked the few yards to the main hospital. A sloping walkway led down to discoloured plastic flap doors. Beyond, the wide basement corridor was cluttered with crates of empty bottles and metal trollies with red rubber mattresses.

The Radiotherapy reception area was also used to store

stacking chairs, trollies and other hospital paraphernalia.

When my name was called, I went through the door in a wooden partition which divided the consultant's office from the rest of the cavernous room. An impatient nurse dragged my jumper over my head, slipped my vest straps off my shoulders and ordered me onto the examination couch. Only then did the consultant turn round from his desk under the high, green, whitewashed window and without uttering a word, marked four ink crosses on my front and back with a felt pen. Then, dressed in a striped hospital robe, I was sent back to the waiting area.

Tattered newspaper supplements and posters on the wall were the only distraction from concern about what was going to happen next. One poster declared the danger of cigarettes, the other the importance of breast-screening programmes. Someone had tacked home-made paper chains across the ceiling and dabbed gobbets of cotton wool on the glass-panelled door. Never have Christmas decorations looked so depressing! Eighty minutes later I was given the first dose of X-ray treatment.

In one corner of the barn-like reception area was a cubicle which housed a console of knobs and dials. Beyond the glass observation panel was a brightly lit treatment area. Access to it was by way of a thick lead-lined door emblazoned with scarlet lettering: NO ADMITTANCE EXCEPT BY AUTHORISED PERSONS.

Two young female technicians tugged on the handle and the door swung open with a loud sucking sound. Inside, the room was dominated by the X-ray machine, a grey metallic praying mantis with multiple glass eyes focused on the trolley beneath.

Against one wall was a table stacked with large and small pillows and a pile of cotton blankets.

The girls quickly positioned me on the trolley for the first treatment. Lying on my 'good' side with pillows to support my back and both arms cradling my head, I was told to keep perfectly still. Then the technicians departed, the thick door thudding into place behind them.

For the next two minutes I lay in this frozen pose, my thoughts racing. Were the villainous cancer cells ducking and dodging down there in my chest as the X-ray heroes hurtled into battle? And who would win possession of my body: the cancer baddies or the radiotherapy goodies? Then the girls returned to re-arrange the battle area.

This time I lay on my back, little beanbags piled on my chest around the ink cross target area. Apparently these bags were filled with seeds called Lincoln Bolus which conveniently absorbed any radiation that might otherwise stray into no-man's-land.

In physical terms it was a painless exercise. The machine silently treated the disease while, like figures on a silent cinema screen, the technicians carried on an animated conversation from behind the safety of the glass observation panel. Twice more I was re-positioned and then it was back to the hostel to while away the long hours until the next treatment session.

Morale at the hostel appeared to be quite high. Even those who were suffering unpleasant side-effects tried to laugh them off. We sat, chatted and drank cups of instant coffee or snacked on crisps and chocolates brought in by visitors. But I suspected that if the way I felt was anything to go by, this cheerfulness was no more than a façade for a multitude of seething anxieties. Except, that is, for one patient who really seemed to be genuinely enjoying the whole wretched business.

May was in her late 30s, the sort of woman who melted into the background. Her figure was small and shapeless, her mouse-coloured hair permed into neat waves around her pale face.

Eventually I heard her story.

Upon leaving school at 14, May went to work as a check-out girl in a small family supermarket and had remained in the same job ever since. Every August she and her widowed mother went by coach to Skegness for two weeks. Otherwise all May did was go to and from home to the shop.

She had no social life, wasn't interested in clothes and was what the rest of her workmates described as someone who 'liked to keep herself to herself'. Believing that there was nothing she could do to alter her humdrum lifestyle, May accepted it. Then she got cancer and overnight everything changed.

Whilst in hospital May's workmates showered her with 'get well' cards and gifts. Customers she only knew by sight turned up to visit her and, suddenly the centre of attention, May blossomed like the desert after rain.

'Having cancer has been the most exciting thing that's ever happened to me,' May assured me, adding, 'One of the girls at the shop has promised to take me shopping for some trendy gear and I'm going to join a Singles Club. I never knew I had so many friends and I've got cancer to thank for that!'

If cancer could prompt someone to start enjoying life, it might appear to be a godsend. Unfortunately it was not a reaction likely to enhance May's chances of a good recovery. If cancer gained her the kind of attention she didn't normally attract it was very possible that this lady would value the advantages of staying ill.

If the days at the hostel were tedious the nights were interminable. Around nine each evening an auxiliary brought hot drinks and close behind came Sister with a tray of prettily coloured pills, all liberally distributed and unquestioningly swallowed. Then it was upstairs to bed in the bleak rooms with scored check tiles on the floor and iron bedsteads with hand-knitted harlequin covers.

Lying in the darkness it was always foreboding not sleep which lurked behind closed eyelids. The sharp pinching pain in my left armpit reminded me that I was now a cancer patient. There was no escaping this distinction. In future whatever I did, wherever I went there would always be this persistently nagging fear in the back of my mind; what if 'it' should recur?

The woman in the next bed always talked herself to sleep, endlessly reviewing the medical disasters which had littered her life. Throughout each night the elderly woman by the window made frequent visits to the bathroom, noisily searching for her slippers before groping for the switch by the door. After each expedition she collapsed back into bed and the sound of her struggled breathing kept us awake.

'You ought to ask for a bed downstairs,' my talkative neighbour frequently suggested.

'Oh no,' came the gasping reply. 'They keep those for people who are in a really bad way.'

After 15 visits to the X-ray department, the surface skin on my chest and back became inflamed. Ten days later it had all peeled off. Hair never again grew in my left armpit and my chest felt strangely 'wooden'.

At the time, I had no idea that even in 1978 there was considerable expert evidence around to indicate the long-term dangers of both radiotherapy as a treatment for cancer and other forms of X-ray exposure.

Radiation Risks

Radiotherapy and cytotoxics (chemicals that poison cells) can shrink benign as well as malignant tumours when the cancer cells are still differentiated. That is, when the tumours still retain microscopic traces of their original metabolic function. When tumours are advanced to a point when they are 'undifferentiated', they are highly resistant to X-ray therapy. In fact irradiation in these cases probably *increases* the number of malignant cells in the tumour. (B.C. Schmidt of the Sloane-Kettering Cancer Centre, USA.)

Theoretically, radiotherapy achieves the same objective as surgery. Surgery cuts out the cancer, radiotherapy burns it out. The problem with all X-ray exposure is that it is cumulative. Small doses of X-ray given at intervals over a long period eventually add up to the same as one large dose, and it is difficult to predict what the delayed side-effects of this might eventually be.

The development of the electron microscope enables scientists to observe that radiation causes disruptions in the cell's control mechanism or DNA. Cells damaged in this way are unable to reproduce normally and become malignant. Some researchers even go so far as to claim that radiation activates viral genes in healthy cells which then triggers off malignancy.

Irradiation of certain glands in the body – the thyroid especially – can produce biochemical changes which pave the way for the appearance of disease years afterwards. The classic example of this is what happened to the survivors of Hiroshima and Nagasaki. Twenty and 30 years after these A-bomb explosions, survivors were still developing and dying of leukemia and giving birth to malformed children.

Then there was the Hollywood film crew who were filming on location in Utah not long after the experimental H-bomb explosion in 1954. This provides another powerful example of delayed reaction to powerful radiation. By 1980 46 out of the crew of 220, had died of cancer, including John Wayne, Susan Hayward and Dick Powell. Moreover, at least three of the stars' children also developed cancer.

The plight of the film crew is well documented. What happened to the citizens of the nearby town of Saint George, Utah, has not been so widely publicised, perhaps because nobody linked the extraordinarily high local incidence of cancer with the H-bomb testing in the 1950s. Even today traces of radioactivity can be found in the milk which comes from this farming area.

X-ray treatment for cancer might turn out to be equally as dangerous in the long-term. There are many studies which indicate that radiotherapy causes more trouble than it alleviates when used in any way other than as a palliative. That is, to deaden pain in the terminal stages of cancer when the patient isn't expected to survive long.

The radiotherapy which I had was supposed to 'mop up' the possible spread of cancer cells. In three weeks I was given 3,500 rems. The recommended maximum safety level for those working in X-ray departments is five rems over a period of one year. But as it was pointed out when I requested to know the exact amount of irradiation exposure given to me, cancer patients are special cases. The same safety regulations do not apply and consultants are entitled to take 'justifiable risks' on behalf of the cancer patient without explaining what these risks entail.

In retrospect, if at the time the facts had been explained before I had my course of radiotherapy, I feel sure that my reaction would have been the same as for the advisability of separating the biopsy from more extensive surgery. Informed of the possible long-term effects of post-operative X-ray treatment, I would have elected to leave well alone until there was something definite to treat.

In the light of what I now know about the way correct nutrition can strengthen natural body defences against cancer, I most certainly would not have had radiotherapy at all. Sadly, this is to be wise after the event.

As to the considered opinion of consultants that patients are not able to make reasonable judgements about radiotherapy and must trust the experts to do so for them, if the track record of the 'experts' is a reflection of their 'expertise', surely the survival rate for breast cancer would have improved in the last 30 years? It has remained the same.

The scientific justification for using X-ray treatment on one group of patients and not on another in order to compare long-term results, also seems unfair if the women used in these trials are not informed about the possible long-term risks.

In 1971 King's College Hospital in London studied the long-term effects of X-ray treatment on 2,000 women who had had surgery for breast cancer. Half were given post-operative X-ray treatment and half were not.

At the end of ten years the women who had the irradiation have suffered fewer recurrences than those who did *not* get the treatment. Where King's College is concerned, this provides the justification for post-operative irradiation for breast-cancer patients.

Similar trials were undertaken at the Christie Hospital in Manchester and it was also concluded that although post-operative irradiation didn't change the overall mortality rate, in the short term it did reduce the appearance of 'secondary' growths. However, the average amount of irradiation given at the Christie was much greater than the X-ray doses given to the women in the King's College trials. So what does any of this prove?

To confuse the issue even further, other cancer centres around the world have reported contradictory results declaring that while X-ray therapy may indeed reduce local recurrence of cancer so that more women given this treatment will be alive five years later, the survival rates after ten years show that irradiated women do not fare so well.

As Rose Kushner writes in her well-researched book *Breast Cancer* (1975):

> Increased incidence of skin, bone, lung and liver metastases have appeared in those women *who did receive* radiotherapy, compared to the *control group who did not.*
>
> Since the 1960s there's been a steady flow of research reports (outside the UK) which insist that the long-term risks of radiotherapy treatment for post-operative breast cancer ought to make this treatment obsolete [my italics].

In 1975 Dr Jan Stjernesward of the Swiss Institute for Experimental Cancer Research, seriously questioned the routine use of irradiation after mastectomy and publicly stated: 'In six controlled studies, survival rates were significantly lower amongst women who were irradiated than amongst those who were treated with surgery alone. Stopping the routine use of prophylactic, local radiotherapy could increase survival rates.'

Experts continue to argue. One gives the 'treatment' another doesn't. One hospital gives more, another less, another none at all. All are firmly convinced that according to the scientific evidence they subscribe to, their actions are justified.

Nutrition and X-Ray Side-Effects

It is known that X-ray treatment destroys Vitamins A, C, E, and K in the body, several B Vitamins and essential fatty acids. (And Vitamin C is the anti-stress food factor.) In her book *Getting Well Again* Adele Davies, the highly respected American nutritionist, states: 'Many harmful substances are formed in the body by the destruction of malignant tissue (by X-ray or chemotherapy) and the liver will more readily do its work of detoxification if Vitamin C and Vitamin E are generously supplied. This helps prevent skin burning, pain and scarring.'

In 1966 in the USA, 54 women suffering from cancer of the cervix went for irradiation treatment. One week beforehand half were given a diet rich in Vitamin A and other nutrients. Three weeks after completion of treatment, 63 per cent of the group which did not have the diet showed a favourable response to treatment. Sixty three per cent was the expected average response. But the women who had been on the diet showed a favourable response rate of 97 per cent or more than 30 per cent above average. (George E. Berkley, 'Cancer: How to Prevent It and How to Help Your Doctor Fight It', PhD, 1978.)

So far as I know, even offering these harmless food factors to patients before they undergo a course of radiotherapy is not routine practice. Not yet.

Chemotherapy

This third 'standard practice' procedure in the armoury of orthodox cancer treatments dates back to 1943, when in the last war the American Liberty Ship the *John E. Harvey* sank with a hundred tons of mustard gas on board. (The fact that this war-weapon was outlawed by all combatants who signed the Geneva Convention, is beside the point!)

It was noted that those seamen who were pulled out of the

water alive, suffered a marked decrease in leukocytes (white blood cells). This lead to laboratory experiments on rats with induced leukemia (cancer of the blood) to see if mustard-gas derivatives could retard the fatal proliferation of white blood cells in this type of cancer.

Promising results (with rats) prompted drug houses to begin searching for other poisonous substances which might have an anti-cancer effect. Since 1946 dozens of cellular poisons (called cytotoxics) have been developed for use against human cancers.

These drugs are taken orally, injected, or infused directly into a vein over a period of hours. Once described by the eminent British oncologist Sir Stanford Cole as the treatment of last resort, the side-effects of chemotherapy invariably have drastic effects on the patient.

In the absence of skilled counselling to improve his morale, or special diets to help cleanse the toxins from his body, the patient is involved in a treatment which is often worse than the symptoms of the disease itself.

Theoretically, the chemicals used are supposed to destroy fast-dividing cell structures, cancer tumours usully coming into this category. Unfortunately the drugs are not selective and also destroy fast-dividing healthy cells.

One patient in ten may gain some extension of life given this treatment, but the price paid is high. Four out of five patients will suffer from any or all of the following reactions: loss of hair; vomiting; mouth ulceration; constipation; abdominal pain; and anorexia, as well as many other debilitating side-effects. There is a school of thought amongst cancer specialists that chemotherapy would be more effective if given before radiotherapy – even before surgery – but not as a last resort.

In his book *Conquering Cancer*, Dr Lucien Israel maintains that diseased cells are rendered highly resistant to cytotoxic drugs by irradiation. Certainly the success rate for this treatment would indicate that introducing poisonous substances into a patient already seriously ill, is hardly justified. As with other orthodox approaches to cancer, chemotherapy has not changed the overall mortality rates for this disease in the past three decades. Yet it seems that doctors who have nothing more to offer the seriously-ill patient would rather give some form of treatment than none at all.

Dr Victor Richards, in his book *The Wayward Cell, Cancer* observed that in the States chemotherapy was primarily used to keep the patient returning for treatment and goes on to say:

> ... chemotherapy serves an extremely valuable role in keeping patients oriented towards proper medical therapy and prevents the feeling of being abandoned by the physicians ... Judicious employment and the screening of potentially useful drugs (cytotoxics) may also *prevent the spread of cancer quackery.* (emphasis added)

In other words, chemotherapy is not only a 'last resort' treatment, but one which will prevent patients looking elsewhere for less harsh treatments!

At best, treating cancer symptoms with chemotherapy means the patient is going to feel a lot worse before feeling any better, and because cytotoxic drugs all depress the body's natural defence system, the patient becomes extremely vulnerable to other infections. Even catching an ordinary cold can be a major setback.

'Chemotherapy is unpleasant for the patient however well it is supervised,' says Patricia Downie, author of *Cancer Rehabilitation*. 'From the point of view of nutrition, effects on the intestine may well result in malabsorption of nutrients. Better nourished patients are able to withstand higher doses of drugs.' In Glasgow Professor Kenneth Calman has demonstrated that Vitamin A (fresh carrots and fish-liver oil being two rich sources) is a biological necessity for healthy human cell growth. He found that cancer patients were notoriously deficient in Vitamin A. Patients at his Glasgow hospital were given chemotherapy *and* large doses of Vitamin A and responded to treatment much better than those patients with low levels of this vitamin in their blood.

Both X-ray and chemotherapy treatment disrupts body chemistry by leeching health-giving vitamins from the system. In order to function efficiently even a healthy person's immune system needs a diet rich in essential nutrients and vitamin supplements. What happens when the cancer patient is subjected to prolonged and aggressive treatments without this nutritional consideration is not hard to imagine.

Sound nutrition is common sense, yet the standard of food given to the residents of the Radiotherapy hostel where I stayed was pitiful – especially when compared to the diets given at the Bristol Centre.

It seemed important that somewhere in this book about gentle therapies for cancer control, readers should be given the facts about the way orthodox cancer specialists approach the management of cancer. It is an approach which has changed little in the last 30 years. Fear, pain and a sense of helplessness are too often the depressing accompaniments to cancer, the chronic illness which now effects one in four people in the UK each year.

If I've painted a harsh picture of orthodox therapies this is because it is drawn from personal experience at a time when reliable information about gentle therapies was not available to me. Like my fellow patients, I did not question whether or not we were getting the best available treatment. I just accepted it.

When I set out to write this book I felt it wouldn't be fair to saddle readers with 'either/or' decisions. There's enough stress associated with having cancer without adding to it. But the beauty of the gentle therapies is that because they are harmless, they can be valuable complementary methods for patients already having orthodox treatments once you know how to incorporate them into your daily routine.

The wholistic therapies which form The Gentle Way may sound like new ideas for those who have not come across them before. The techniques involved are not new. They have been researched and used for more than ten years, principally in the USA but almost always as *separate* methods for treating cancer with natural measures.

People have used the nutritional therapies or they have used the non-physical approach which involves autogenic training or they have tried the vigorous form of metabolic therapy which includes injections of laetrile and enzymes, and other vitamins and minerals which discourage malignant tumours. And because in the past people have used either one or the other of these natural ways for cancer control, in the chapters which follow I have described them separately. But it is a combination of these effective methods which comprises the wholistic approach as used at Bristol. And it is this combined approach which cleanses the whole system and prepares the gentle way for recovery.

There are many stories about the way our thoughts can influence physical health. The following is a favourite of mine.

A young man fell in love. Every week he liked to give his girl a big bunch of red roses which were her favourite flowers. Unfortunately the love affair didn't last. The girl met and married someone else.

The young man was heartbroken. Not long afterwards he was invited to have dinner with friends and the table centrepiece happened to be a bowl of red rosebuds. To the dismay of the other guests, the young man suffered a bad attack of asthma.

Thereafter he found that whenever he went anywhere near roses, the same thing happened. He was treated with all the usual remedies but nothing happened. He was not allergic to pollen. Eventually his GP sent him to a psychologist who tried to get the young man to understand that because he associated roses with unhappiness, his mind was causing the physical symptoms of 'distress'. Naturally enough, the patient refused to believe he was actually responsible for his own suffering. He 'knew' he was allergic to roses. So the psychologist devised a way to convince him.

When next the young man went for a consultation he was appalled to see on the doctor's desk a bowl of roses. He promptly collapsed, gasping for air. When he was finally able to speak again he looked accusingly at his doctor and wheezed: 'How could you put roses in here when you knew what would hapen?' With a smile, the psychologist pulled a rose from the vase and thrust it at his patient.

The rose was made of plastic, the young man was cured.

That something as serious as cancer has its origins in the mind of the patient may seem like a wild oversimplification.

But this is not a new concept.

As far back as the second century AD eminent physicians were observing this. Galen was one of them. This medical authority of the day noticed that 'melancholic women were more prone to cancer than their sanguine sisters'.

The medical literature of the 18th and 19th centuries is littered with similar observations. Negative emotions were often the precursor of physical disease.

In 1701 a certain Doctor Gendron wrote the following: 'Mrs Emerson, upon the death of her daughter, underwent great affliction and perceived her breast to swell which soon after grew painful. At last it broke out in a most inveterate cancer which consumed a great part of it in a short time. She had always enjoyed perfect health before her grievous family loss.'

This physician noticed that the shock of bereavement often triggered the onset of cancer in certain of his patients.

In 1846 the following passage appeared in a book called *The Nature and Treatment of Cancer* which again points out the connection between mind and cancer but takes this concept an important step further.

> Much has been written on the influence of mental misery, sudden reverses of fortunes and habitual gloominess of temper on the deposition of carcinomatous matter, which would seem to constitute the most powerful cause of the disease. Morbid emotions produce defective innervation and this causes a perversion of nutrition which in turn causes the formation of carcinoma.
>
> Although the influence of mental disquietude has never been made a matter for demonstration, it would be vain to deny facts of a very convincing character in respect to the agency of the mind in the production of this disease. I have met with cases in which the connection appeared so clear that to question its reality would have seemed to struggle against reason.

One hundred and thirty six years ago this Victorian physician had put his finger on the psychobiological route to the illness we call cancer. In other words, what goes on in the minds of certain people has a direct bearing on their physical health.

Psychobiological Studies

Current research has already described the interaction between emotions and the chemical changes which take place in the body. (S. Greer and P.M. Silberfarb, *Psychological Medicine*, 1982.)

When someone becomes psychologically disturbed it is possible to measure the chemical changes which occur.

A study of women with breast cancer showed that those who had a good psychological response to their disease had substantially higher levels of gamma globulin in their blood which is the serum the body produces to build up the antibodies which combat infection and disease.

It would follow that if a woman with a poor response could be helped to alter her attitude of pessimism to one of optimism, then she would be able to enjoy the protection of extra gamma globulin too. Unfortunately, the cosy exercise of proving theories is often far removed from clinical practice.

'Future studies,' Dr Greer writes, 'will need to be based on more sophisticated techniques for measuring biological as well as psychological variables. Of critical importance for psychological studies of cancer are advances in our understanding of the neuro-endocrine control of the immune system.'

While scientists dabble with imponderables, the big question is, can cancer patients exercise any degree of control over this mysterious biochemical system? The short answer is 'yes'. We do so every moment of our lives, but not always to our best advantage if our responses to what goes on around us triggers negative chemical changes in our bodies.

When we feed negative thought patterns into the nervous

system we unwittingly set in motion a series of reactions which create the conditions for disease. The techniques for reversing this process can be learned once we understand – and believe – that the brain is not just the seat of consciousness and intelligence but a power house for the production or suppression of many complex chemicals which have a direct bearing on personal well-being.

You don't have to know what these chemicals are – or the complicated workings of your own anatomy – in order to learn techniques which will control this *natural* ebb and flow of internal energies. Leave that to the researchers.

Everyone has heard of psychosomatic illnesses. GPs are recorded as saying that as many as 60 per cent of people coming to their surgeries complain of ailments which can't be accounted for in physical terms and do not respond to ordinary medication. These are what have been called 'stress-related illnesses'. When unresolved stress curdles body chemistry then the victim becomes the unwitting architect of his own disease.

Unresolved stress is interpreted by the brain as 'a threat to survival'. This prompts the body to protect itself. It does this by automatically releasing into the system the chemical which will power the body to escape from the threat. In primitive man this was either to beat a hasty retreat or stand and fight.

Today neither is socially acceptable. Even when his mind tells him he is under threat, the average citizen doesn't abandon his obligations and head for the hills. So the hormones (adrenalin and steroids) which have been released into the bloodstream in order to promote direct action are not used and remain to circulate and disrupt the delicate chemical balance of the entire natural defence system.

In particular, over a long period suppressed stress interferes with the production of T-lymphocytes which are programmed to combat disease.

Duodenal ulcers provide a classic example of an illness which begins in the mind but ends up as an acute physical problem. And treating the symptoms of such a disease does not tackle the root cause of the problem. This can only be accomplished by treating the sick person on every level of his 'being'.

People are not just physical beings. Health is not a closed-circuit system. Health is a subtle blend and balance of mental, spiritual and physical ease in compatible surroundings. The way we behave, the way we think either enhances or sabotages our intrinsic well-being.

And just as people who get ulcers tend to conform to a particular personality pattern, so are there definite fundamental characteristics which apply to people who are susceptible to the disease of cancer.

The Cancer Personality

That people who get cancer share similar life histories and personality traits was clearly established by the American psychologist Lawrence LeShan. (L. LeShan, *You Can Fight for Your Life*, 1977.)

For more than ten years LeShan amassed a vast amount of material gleaned from hundreds of personal interviews with cancer patients and scrutiny of written case histories of thousands more. And as well as talking to cancer patients, LeShan made a point of talking to their families in order to collect all the factors which would construct a picture of 'the person most likely to get cancer'.

As a control to these studies, LeShan also examined the case histories and personalities of patients with other chronic diseases.

At the end of two years, LeShan had isolated a number of common denominators which only applied to cancer patients, but to test his hypothesis he instructed a colleague to assemble a collection of personal case histories composed of cancer patients mixed up with patients suffering from other complaints.

LeShan was able to pick out the cancer patients from the others with 80 per cent accuracy.

A patient called Catherine was a typical example of the kind of person LeShan found to be a candidate for cancer.

As a child Catherine had felt rejected and unloved in a home where the intellectual mother dominated the household and the father was a somewhat weak individual. He also regarded any physical contact with either of his daughters as repugnant.

Catherine's sister was an attractive extrovert. Catherine was just the opposite. When her sister always managed to claim more parental attention than she did, Catherine retreated into her shell, believing that this was because she was basically an unlikeable person. The only consolation she had was in her love of music.

When she was old enough for college, Catherine left home to live with fellow students and study music. Concentrating on her studies and beginning to enjoy a normal social life as well, she was at last happy. Then her puritanical father decided that city life was exposing her to moral dangers and insisted Catherine enrol in a college nearer to home.

From then on she lost interest in music and when she met a man her mother approved of, Catherine married him.

They had four children and although Catherine tried to keep up with local musical activities, she found herself immersed in boring domesticity. Her health began to suffer. She felt overwhelmed by a sense of failure and the fact that she could not seem to get much affection from her husband. She decided that she was never going to be able to get much enjoyment from living. At this point Catherine developed cancer.

In the course of his research, LeShan interviewed hundreds of cancer patients. Again and again the same life pattern was repeated.

Adverse childhood events leading to
Early sense of inadequacy

Lack of satisfactory parental relationships
A poor outlet for creative energy
Inability to vent emotions
A defeatist attitude towards their own endeavours
Stoical acceptance of failure and/or misfortune when it occurred

But there was still one additional common factor which invariably heralded the first symptoms of cancer. This, LeShan found, was the loss of an important relationship such as divorce or desertion, followed by depression.

Studies made elsewhere in the 1960s and 70s, and mostly in the United States, also show that cancer patients share other denominators which make them likely candidates for the disease.

Lung cancer patients, it has been found, not only tend to be heavy smokers but tend to smoke more at night.

A consistent factor in cases of breast cancer is the woman's inability to suckle her children.

Women with cervical cancer share a strong sex-drive but find it difficult to achieve orgasm due to rigid inhibitions about self-control.

As for cancer of the prostrate, apparently this is found more frequently in older men who make a habit of foreplay which does not culminate in sexual intercourse.

Sexual inhibitions (which are also part of the pattern which goes to make up the 'cancer personality') that suppress organ function increase susceptibility to disease in the reproductive system.

The psychological factors which make one person more vulnerable to ulcers or another to cancer are deeply ingrained. But if the problems lie within, so do the answers. With the right kind of guidance, patients can learn exercises which will stimulate the nervous system to convey healing messages to the physical body. And we are not referring to a new-fangled procedure but to the ancient practice of meditation. The only new part to this gentle cancer control therapy is the guided imagery techniques which accompany the relaxation and meditation exercises taught at the Bristol Cancer Help Centre. These are based on the work of Eastern traditional medicine, Ainslie Meares and Carl Simonton.

Unknown Factors

Carl Simonton trained as a radiotherapist but soon became disillusioned by a form of cancer treatment which left no room for imaginative innovation. Time and again the same treatments were prescribed and repeatedly the overall results were disappointing. But what could a young doctor do? He'd been taught orthodox methods of cancer management and apart from surgery, radiotherapy and drug remedies there was nothing else to offer patients.

Then in 1969 Simonton happened to hear a lecture given by a prominent immunotherapist. This man talked about the new theory that everyone has cancer many times during his or her lifetime but never knows it. He believed that there were two basic factors which allowed cancer cells to form tumours.

First, some cancer cells develop a strong resistance to elimination by the body's normal defence system. Secondly, the defence system somehow becomes inefficient and does not recognise the abnormal cells as harmful matter.

The immunologist then described how he had taken patients suffering from terminal leukemia (blood cancer) and made a solution of a concentrate of their abnormal white blood cells. He then applied this to the patient's skin hoping to produce an 'immune response'.

(This is the principle involved in vaccination for small-pox. The small-pox virus is weakened so although it can't produce disease in the vaccinated person it will stimulate that person's immune system to make specific antibodies which will instantly recognise and destroy any subsequent small-pox infection.)

The immunologist's experiment with his leukemic patients produced remarkable results. Half of them went into remission. The scientist promptly published this experiment and others tried to duplicate it – with disappointing results.

When Simonton heard this it occurred to him that what was lacking in the repeat experiments with leukemic patients was the enthusiasm generated by the immunologist who had taken considerable trouble to explain to his cancer patients and their families exactly what he was hoping to achieve. Simonton felt that this had something to do with the initial successes. It seemed to him that there were unknown factors at work which could not be measured scientifically – or repeated by other investigators.

Another area of cancer care which attracted Simonton was that of spontaneous regression. Despite a very unfavourable prognosis, a small number of his patients did make unexpected recoveries. Simonton set out to find if there was a common denominator amongst them and almost immediately found one.

In every case history of patients who had recovered despite the odds against them, it was the attitude of the patient towards life which emerged as the shared factor.

Excited by this discovery, Simonton wondered if it might be possible to teach this positive attitude to other less well motivated cancer patients to influence their chances of recovery.

The mind-over-matter techniques which Carl Simonton and his wife Stephanie pioneered in Texas in the 1970s, form a good illustration of the basis for the non-physical aspects of the therapies used at Bristol.

Mind Control

In his clinical work with cancer patients, Simonton asked a selected few to learn what he called 'mental imagery' exercises.

Simonton's first patient was a 61 year old man with extensive throat cancer. He was emaciated, could hardly swallow his own saliva and close to death.

After explaining how cancer had managed to evade his immune system and form the tumour and how radiotherapy would help destroy it, Simonton taught this patient how to achieve a state of deep physical relaxation. Then he asked the man to make a mental picture of his cancer tumour and how the radiation was overcoming it. He was also asked to practise this exercise several times a day at home.

A year and a half later the man was not only alive but cancer free. And amazingly, it wasn't only the cancer which this patient managed to overcome with these mind control techniques. He also rid himself of arthritis and the impotence which had plagued him for more than 20 years.

Over the next decade, Carl Simonton and his wife Stephanie who is a psychotherapist, combined the conventional cancer treatment of radiotherapy with this mind-over-matter approach to generate self-healing. Gradually, they amassed a treasure-trove of clinical observations to confirm the value of what was then and to a certain extent still is today, 'unorthodox' therapy.

The Simontons found that, in general, patients with negative attitudes towards life had a poor response to treatment compared with those who had an optimistic outlook. When the poor responders were helped, with psychotherapy, to readjust their thinking, they also started to improve.

One case was of particular interest to the Simontons. This was a 35 year old woman who had a cancerous wound on the cervix which was causing widespread infection. The outlook for this patient was extremely poor.

Simonton treated her with radiotherapy and nothing else. Two weeks later the tumour had regressed to half its original size. Somewhat puzzled, Simonton asked the woman if she'd any idea why this might have happened. She replied that perhaps it was due to the four glasses of grape juice which she drank daily.

As she was obviously responding well to irradiation, Simonton decided to explain his mental-imaging exercises to see if the patient would like to co-operate.

'That sounds like meditation,' the woman exclaimed. Simonton agreed that this was fair comment and asked why she'd made it. Her answer was that she'd recently come across a book by the healer Edgar Cayce and decided to try regular daily meditation. When Simonton asked her why she hadn't mentioned this before, the woman admitted that she felt sure an orthodox doctor would only ridicule her for trying it!

The pioneer work of the Simontons in the field of cancer therapy is the subject of their book *Getting Well Again*, a publication which has gained them deserved respect in both medical and lay circles. At the University of California this book is now required reading for students of experiential psychology. In the UK however, the work of the Simontons and LeShan has stirred minimal professional interest.

There is one last story from the work of the Simontons which highlights the need for psychotherapy before mental imagery if these exercises are to be used effectively by the cancer patient.

This Simonton patient was 19, a youngster with a two-year history of Hodgkin's Disease (cancer of the lymphatic glands). When he was brought to Simonton he was near to death and knew it. But Simonton realised that when a patient had given up all hope of living sometimes the resistance to mental imagery techniques was greatly reduced and therefore more effective.

This young patient was no exception. After several imaging sessions there was a rapid change for the better and he was sent home. A week later he was re-admitted and again very ill.

Simonton suggested that if he sincerely wanted to get well, the young man would have persevered with the exercises. The patient replied that he couldn't see himself well again.

Delving into his past history, Simonton learned that in

childhood this patient had a younger brother who had a kidney complaint. He had gained all the parental attention and love.

It transpired that the young man found his cancer got him the sympathy and attention which he was lacking in his earlier life.

'If I could just stay moderately sick and not severely ill, that would be fine,' he admitted.

For such patients the mental imagery exercises are of no use until they are helped to appreciate the deeper reasons for their cancer. Patients like Simonton's young man and like May, my fellow patient at the Radiotherapy Hostel, were severely handicapped by emotional factors they didn't realise would impede their chance of proper recovery. Both needed their cancer in order to attract the love and attention which they both craved but could not get when they were healthy. This is what psychologists call 'secondary gain', a complication which cannot be appreciated by the patient, let alone overcome unless skilled counselling is available.

That cancer is the physical symptom of deeply repressed hostility is another fact which many patients are unable to face up to without psychotherapeutic help. Then again, for some, cancer is a means of committing suicide, a kind of escape from unresolved emotional conflicts which have subconsciously become intolerable. Then the cancer patient needs the lifeline afforded by skilled counselling. In the words of the poet Thornton Wilder: '... despair probes the organs one by one, seeking the easiest entrance for the kill ...'

At present there are only a very few hospitals in the UK where nurses have been trained to counsel cancer patients. One of them is the University Hospital in South Manchester in a scheme set up by Dr Peter Maguire after a three-year study of the emotional needs of cancer patients. Maguire has been able to show that patients who receive counselling on average make a better recovery than those who don't although long-term results have yet to be assessed.

Hidden Forces

In every cancer patient there is a very large – if hidden – fund of courage and resolution which needs to be harnessed in the fight for recovery. It is the same vital force which exists in every human who achieves some apparently superhuman endeavour.

Sometimes this force is pure aggression, as with sportsmen pushing themselves to the limits of endurance. At other times the hidden factor is generated by quiet determination. Two excellent examples of people who have – perhaps unwittingly – tapped this hidden force to reverse otherwise unfavourable cancer prognoses are the Lancashire journalist Pat Seed MBE and Bob Champion, the National Hunt jockey.

In 1976 when Pat Seed was told she had only a short time to live, she set out to raise 3 million pounds for a CAT scanner for the Christie Hospital in Manchester where she was undergoing treatment. Not only did this remarkable woman achieve her target, but despite the physical effort required to tour the countryside and promote the fund-raising campaign, by the time the scanner was installed Pat Seed's cancer was in remission. It remained so until the tragic death of her husband in the Abbeystead waterworks explosion early in 1984, when she suffered a relapse and died in August of the same year.

As for Bob Champion, his recovery from cancer began when he set himself the goal of riding the 1981 Derby winner. Again, perhaps unconsciously, he set in motion that indefinable psychological factor which can reverse the course of physical disease.

So if these hidden factors can be deliberately set in motion by the informed cancer patient, what a difference this would make to the fight for recovery!

The story of a young American psychologist called Neil Fiore illustrates what can be achieved by the cancer patient who cultivates the correct mental attitude towards his treatment.

A staunch believer in meditation and jogging to relax the body and clear the mind, when Neil Fiore found that he had cancer of the scrotum with secondaries in one lung, although he elected to have whatever treatments his doctors advised he also realised that whatever they did would be directed at killing the cancer and not at him as the whole person who had become sick. So he decided to add his personal resources to the treatments.

Each time he had chemotherapy he created a mental picture of what was happening in his body. He imagined the 'confused' cancer cells, then he pictured hordes of muscular white blood cells tracking down and destroying them.

Every week for seven months Neil went for injections and suffered all the pain and fear which accompanies this treatment. He continued to steel himself to regard the drugs as 'powerful allies' fighting alongside his own healthy white cells. Between times, he worked hard at keeping his mind and body in peak condition, using his own meditation and mental imagery exercises and to reduce worry and tension he also kept up daily jogging sessions.

In the Autumn of that same year, the cancer in Neil's lung had gone. He'd lost all his hair which made him depressed and then he developed a high fever which sent him back to hospital. The chemotherapy treatments had to be suspended and immediately he started to improve.

Today Neil Fiore insists that he feels healthier than before the illness which taught him to generate that mysterious 'X' factor in his fight for recovery.

In a recording of his experience made to help other patients, Neil says: 'You have the right to question your doctor. If you are worried or in conflict about a procedure, ask his reasons for recommending it. Ask about alternative methods.

'Don't waste energy worrying. Don't delegate responsibility for your life to your doctor and force him to play God. Respect your doctor's opinion but respect also your own body and judgement. Above all, never lose hope ...'

In the last five years two UK hospital psychology

departments have been studying the value of psychotherapy for patients with breast cancer.

Dr Steven Greer, a psychologist at King's College Hospital in London has come up with the same observations which LeShan and the Simontons made ten years ago.

The following are quotations from the scientific paper *Psychological Medicine* which was published in 1982.

> ... the patient group who had the most favourable outcome differed strikingly from all others in its high proportion of individuals who had strong hostile drives without the loss of emotional control. This personality is the antithesis of the 'hopeless' or 'giving up' reaction.
>
> ... long survivors had closer personal relationships, suffered less emotional distress, regarded their physicians as more helpful, complained less and coped better with illness-related problems than was the case amongst short survivors ...

One can only hope that what Dr Greer was observing was not the façade which some patients seem able to erect as a cover to very deep emotional disquietude. Dr Peter Maguire who has been conducting similar studies at University Hospital, South Manchester found that:

> ... patients perceived nurses as being very busy and responsible people (these were nurses trained to counsel cancer patients). They felt that they should not burden them with their worries.
>
> The overall impression gained was that most patients strived hard to maintain the appearance that they were coping well even when this was patently not so. They did so ... to protect both nursing staff and their close relatives from further strain. By doing this they were also protecting themselves from mental suffering.

In 1980 the magazine *Nursing Mirror* published an article written by Dr Peter Maguire and the two nurses who head his research team in Manchester. Again this was concerned with breast cancer patients and was entitled 'A Conspiracy to Pretend that Cancer Patients Cope Emotionally'. The following is an excerpt from this article.

Cancers still cause much suffering and many deaths. So it is inevitable that cancer patients fear that they may suffer terrible pain, waste away and die before their hopes and goals are realised. Even when cancer has been removed successfully the patient has to live with considerable uncertainty as to whether and when the cancer will recur. Hence, many cancer patients and their relatives experience considerable strain.

The treatments used to combat cancers may greatly intensify this strain because they often have unpleasant consequences. Thus treatment may include the removal of a part of the body which was crucial to the patient's self-esteem ... Radiotherapy and chemotherapy commonly cause fatigue, depression, nausea, vomiting and hair loss. These side effects can be so severe that the patients and relatives come to dread further treatments or even refuse them, particularly when more aggressive regimes of cytotoxic (cell poisoning) drugs are employed.

So it should be expected that some patients and relatives find the strain of living with the cancers and consequences of treatment too much for them and develop serious psychological problems.

Recent studies have found that between 20 per cent and 40 per cent of women who undergo mastectomy for breast cancer develop depressive illness, anxiety neurosis or sexual problems within 12 months of surgery. A similar proportion (23 per cent) of patients who undergo colostomy for ano-rectal cancer develop psychiatric illness. The effect of such surgery on sexual functioning can be catastrophic ...

Few patients or relatives who develop psychological problems appear to get the help they need. This seems largely due to the failure of those concerned with cancer care to establish how the patients and relatives have reacted.

So far these studies have received scant attention from cancer specialists although many nurses who look after cancer patients are already aware of the problems.

Psychotherapy requires the consistent efforts of skilled staff. It also needs a shift of attitude on the part of most oncology departments if it is ever to become an integral part of cancer management.

Performing surgery or switching on a radiotherapy

machine or injecting cytotoxics are straightforward procedures directed at the physical symptoms. Coping with the emotional results of such aggressive measures are more complicated, require much more highly trained staff and are therefore beyond the resources of the NHS, even though it has been clearly shown that giving the cancer patient the best chance of recovery depends upon more than physical treatment.

Fortunately, as so often happens nowadays, once certain health-conscious members of the public became aware of the need, a network of specialist cancer-help support groups were gradually established up and down the country. (NB: These are not to be confused with branches of The Mastectomy Association.)

One of the first to be established was the group at Diss in Norfolk, under the sponsorship of a local GP who had practised medicine in the area for more than thirty years.

For some years before his retirement in 1979, Dr Ian Pearce had recognised that caring for his cancer patients at a purely physical level was not enough. He had also discovered that he possessed the gift of healing.

Once he had researched the work done with cancer patients by the Simontons and LeShan in the USA and Ainslie Meares in Australia, Dr Pearce selected a few of his cancer patients and offered them the chance to learn meditation and visualisation techniques using bio-feedback devices. Quite soon this led to a regular Sunday group in the doctor's home, where cancer patients and close family members could meet together in relaxed surroundings.

As these people were encouraged to talk about themselves and about their illness, emotional problems that might have contributed to their disease – might even be blocking their chances of recovery – started to surface.

Dr Pearce soon began to see the dynamic benefits of this group therapy. Patients who had previously felt isolated by their disease, were able to gain comfort and confidence by talking with others going through the same crisis.

In his book *The Holistic Approach to Cancer*, Dr Pearce

describes the benefits derived by those of his patients who
attend the Diss Cancer Help Group.

'Generally it is found that there is a reduction in the level
of symptoms, such as pain, loss of appetite, lethargy, weight
loss and depression, and a correspondingly reduced
dependence upon analgesics.

'Almost invariably there is a massive change in the
outlook of the patient. This is characterised by the
acceptance of cancer as 'just another illness', a loss of fear –
both of the disease itself and of dying – and a very real
appreciation of the worth of every minute of every day.

'Life becomes no longer something to be dreaded, or the
day to be *got through* but not necessarily enjoyed … there is a
profound healing influence upon the whole family, together
with a breaking down of the barriers which are so often
erected after cancer has been diagnosed.

'This is of the utmost importance to the progress of the
patient …'

When I first met Dr Pearce I was just getting over my
mastectomy and full of fears for the future. The work I saw
being done at Diss transformed my entire outlook on the
nature of cancer and its psychological origins. I saw how
patients enabled to talk openly about cancer were helped to
realign the negative attitudes which had been hindering
recovery. From Dr Pearce I first started to understand how
it was possible to exert the positive emotional attitudes
which could stimulate natural healing mechanisms.

Enlightened physicians like Dr Ian Pearce are not
content to wait for official consent. Dr Pearce now lectures
worldwide on the wholistic (or 'holistic') approach to cancer
management at present denied the average cancer patient
by the medical establishment.

But of course psychological help and counselling are only
one stage of the total approach designed to encourage the
patient to start thinking of himself as more than just a
physical being. Diet, too, must play a co-ordinated part in
the gentle therapy programme.

5   THE FEAR STOPS RIGHT HERE!

How would you like to live where there's no cancer? Perhaps you believe that such a possibility only exists in the realms of wishful thinking. If so, you'd be wrong.

Throughout the world – admittedly nowadays only in remote localities – there live groups of people who do not know the meaning of cancer. From time to time this has attracted the interest of medical observers determined to find out what it is that enables these isolated communities to enjoy a standard of health which for the most part eludes wealthy western civilisations.

These isolated peoples have not found the key to cancer control; it is we who have lost it. And what is this magical formula? Nutrition.

The tiny kingdom of Hunza in North West Pakistan provides a fascinating illustration of this.

Few outsiders attempt the journey to this Himalayan province. The only road is impassible during the winter months and from April to October presents visitors with a treacherous 60 mile bus or jeep ride which is said to loosen the teeth of the most intrepid traveller.

Nevertheless, occasional teams of medical scientists have braved the mountain passes which separate the Shangri-La people of Hunza from the rest of civilisation.

In 1922 the British surgeon and physician Robert McCarrison returned from such an expedition and wrote in the American Medical Association journal: 'the Hunzakuts have no known incidence of cancer. They have abundant crops of apricots which they dry in the sun and use very largely in their food.'

Many readers failed to make the connection between the absence of cancer and apricots, but this information was a fascinating confirmation of the work which was then

occupying the father and son team of researchers in San
Francisco.

Physician Ernst T. Krebs and his biochemist son Dr
Ernst T. Krebs Jnr co-discovered Vitamin B-17 which is
the chemical tag for food factors known as nitrilosides.
What they then knew about B-17 tied in beautifully with
the traditional eating habits of the Hunzakuts which
entitled them to the accolade of the healthiest nation on
earth.

The vital link between cancer and diet is not a new
concept. It is, however, one which is persistently rejected by
conventional physicians despite the wealth of empirical
evidence which has been accumulated over the last two or
three decades, largely due to the crusading efforts of
enlightened physicians and pioneer biochemists like the
Krebses in the United States.

The Krebs' absorbing interest in a nutritional substance
which when left out of the diet paved the way for cancer,
was prompted by the work of Scottish physician John Beard.

The Trophoblast Theory

In 1902 Beard discovered that the body's primary
mechanism for destroying malignant cells was apparently
due to the action of enzymes produced in the pancreas. He
observed that this natural protection was linked to the way
certain cells called trophoblasts behaved, first to make life
possible and then, if allowed to proliferate, by turning
malignant.

The trophoblast cell is the one responsible for burrowing
into the wall of the uterus so that the fertilised egg at
conception can attach itself and take nourishment from the
mother's bloodstream through the placenta. Without this
primitive cell there would be no pregnancy because the
human embryo would starve to death.

Dr Beard found that on the 56th day of pregnancy the

pancreas in the mother's body produces an enzyme called chymotrypsin which switches off the trophoblast cells. Also at the 56th day, the baby's pancreas begins to function.

Having done the work they were designed to do, the trophoblasts were rendered harmless but if for some reason the mother's pancreas failed to produce the switching-off enzyme, disasterous results for both mother and child followed. The action of the rogue trophoblasts, Dr Beard noticed, was exactly the same as the action of other body cells which turning malignant, started to 'eat their way' into healthy tissue.

Dr Beard's studies strongly indicated that cancer is not an unnatural, invasive disease but a serious fault in body chemistry. In the case of the errant trophoblasts, a deficiency or complete lack of the pancreatic enzyme chymotrypsin would cause healthy cells to become cancerous ones. And it is the pancreas which produces a variety of enzymes without which the human digestive system could not metabolise protein in the food we eat.

So at the beginning of this century John Beard was saying that cancer was a deficiency disease. Eighty years on, this learned proposition has done little to deter the orthodox medical profession's determination to treat the symptoms of cancer not the faulty metabolism which allowed disease to form in the first place.

Yet the history of medicine provides many powerful examples of life-threatening ailments turning out to be due to diet deficiencies. The slang name 'Limey' for an Englishman abroad, is one.

When old-time sailing ships went off on long ocean voyages, the crew ate a diet of salt pork. Many died on the high seas, stricken down by a mysterious disease.

These unfortunate sailors haemorrhaged in all the joints of their bodies and their teeth fell out. Then, if they didn't reach land, they died. This disease, dreaded for nearly 200 years, was finally cured when a Navy surgeon instructed every ship to carry supplies of apples and limes. Just by sucking on a lemon the seaman could protect himself against the killer disease of scurvy.

The magic formula was nothing more than Vitamin C.

Pellagra illustrates another diet deficiency disease. In farming areas of the world where maize was the staple food, people often suffered from a form of malnutrition which caused insanity and death. For more than 30 years medical science had no remedy for this terrifying and mysterious illness. Then it was discovered that niacin – one of the B-Vitamins found in yeast and liver – was the miracle answer to so much unnecessary suffering.

This brings us back to the cancer-free people of Hunza and their apricots. What is the connection between this simple fruit and the fact that the Hunzakuts do not suffer from the affliction of cancer which is close to epidemic proportions in civilised countries?

The Hunza people are safely isolated from the rest of the world in their Himalayan valleys. They farm sheep for wool and cultivate apricot orchards without the use of chemical pesticides. When there's a risk of insect damage to the crops, they spray the trees with a mixture of water and ash which seems to do the trick.

Compared to the average western daily diet, the average Hunzakut is a small eater. He eats millet, a range of fresh fruits and vegetables, home-produced honey, other grains and pulses and scarcely any meat. His daily diet totals 1900 calories which includes 50 grammes of vegetable protein and 354 grammes of carbohydrates also obtained from fruit, vegetables and grains.

The average westerner eats 3300 calories daily which contain 100 grammes of meat protein, 157 grammes of fat and 380 grammes of carbohydrates mostly derived from white sugar and refined flour. (Dr Alexander Lead, *National Geographic*, 1973.)

In Hunza 85 is middle-aged and people of over 100 still lead an active life. Two doctors once took a portable cardiograph all the way to Hunza and examined a group of old men whose ages ranged from 90 to 120. They found no evidence of heart disease amongst them, their eyesight was perfect, and most of these people were still putting in a full day's work plus regular games of polo, which is the local form of amusement, *and* going for early morning dips in local glacial rivers.

The doctors were also impressed by the Hunzakuts' strong teeth, thick shining hair and clear complexions.

So what is the secret of so much health and vitality? Apricots! But not just the apricot fruit. The Hunzakuts always crack open the apricot stones and eat the kernels (seeds) as well. In winter they eat dried apricots and press oil from the surplus seeds.

And another question. What is the magic vitamin locked up in the apricot kernel? Vitamin B-17 which is the nitriloside found not only in apricot kernels but in a whole range of foods most of which have either lost favour with the typical westerner's diet or have been stripped of B-17 during manufacturing processes.

So we have the connection between Dr Beard's observations about the anti-cancer enzymes produced in the healthy pancreas and food factors which the pancreas must have if it is to function healthily. Nitrilosides.

Nitrilosides are water soluble food factors found in the seeds of most fruits and in over one-thousand other plants. Wherever isolated groups of 'primitive' people have been found to enjoy exceptionally good health with the absence of malignant and degenerative diseases, study of their eating habits always reveals a high intake of nitriloside-bearing foods. (*Cancer News Journal*, 1970.)

The cereals millet and buckwheat (unprocessed, of course) are rich sources of nitrilosides or Vitamin B-17. So are the sprouts of lentils, mung beans and alfalfa. Beansprouts contain 50 per cent more nitriloside content than the parent plants which is why there is such emphasis on the use of sprouted grains in the Bristol Diet.

Apple pips, the kernels of cherries, peaches, plums, grapes and apricots, are other nourishing sources of B-17 and should always be eaten with the fruit. These fruit seeds also have other health-giving properties. They are rich in

Vitamin A and Vitamin C and natural energy-giving sugars, all vital food factors needed by the immune system if it is successfully to protect the body against disease.

So the widespread western habit of 'spitting out the pips' when eating apples, cherries and the like means that we inadvertently discard the nitrilosides which specifically guard against the formation of cancer.

The Hunzakuts are not the only communities which have naturally protected themselves against chronic debilitating diseases which plague the rest of modern society. There are small pockets of people around the world with widely differing cultural habits but with one shared denominator. These people eat only natural foods.

The Pueblo Indians of New Mexico seldom get cancer or arthritis. They drink a traditional brew made from the ground kernels of cherries, peaches and apricots.

When the American author Robert Houston finished researching the lifestyle of the Pueblos for the book he was writing on cancer prevention, he decided to try making milk-shakes with ground-up apricot kernels.

First he oven-roasted two dozen kernels for ten minutes at 300 degrees, to destroy the enzymes in the seeds which might otherwise upset the stomach if eaten without the whole fruit. Then he put the roasted seeds in an electric blender with a spoonful of honey and half-a-pint (300 ml) of milk.

The drink was so delicious that he drank one every day. After a few days he noticed that two small pink warts which he'd always had on his arm, had turned brown. A day or so later they had become black and at the end of a week of the nitriloside-rich milk-shakes, Houston realised these benign skin blemishes had dropped off leaving clear, healthy skin underneath.

After a life-long study of the value of nitrilosides as a protection against cancer, Dr Krebs Jnr has often publicly announced that cancer is a diet-deficiency disease which occurs when the natural body defences cannot eliminate 'rogue' cells because the food we eat lacks the enzymes richly provided by Vitamin B-17.

Exactly how B-17 works in the body against cancer cells is a complex biochemical mechanism. However, in simplified terms, the following explanation gives a fair idea of what happens when B-17 and cancer cells cross swords. And this reaction depends upon certain biological certainties.

Cancer tissue is always bathed in a fluid containing beta-glucosidase. As soon as this comes into contact with B-17, beta-glucosidase splits the nitriloside molecule into two sugar molecules, one molecule of benzaldehyde and one molecule of hydrogen cyanide. The naturally occurring cyanide in Vitamin B-17 is non-toxic because the body has a built-in ability to neutralise the cyanide molecule if it comes into contact with healthy cells.

Just as the liquid surrounding a cancerous growth is only found at the site of malignant cells, the healthy cell has a liquid partner called rhodanese. Rhodanese instantly combines with cyanide molecules to render them harmless. But the cancer cell does not have rhodanese to protect it so the cyanide molecule released at the site of the tumour certainly can and does attack and poison the cancer tumour. In this way B-17 only harms malignant cells.

Obviously the biochemistry involved is more complex and is fully explained elsewhere.

Some Japanese workers have observed that benzaldehyde alone has an anti-cancer action so possibly the effects of Vitamin B-17 are due to the combined action of cyanide and benzaldehyde – possibly only benzaldehyde if you take into account the recent comments by several researchers which suggest that cyanide being the active principle of Vitamin B-17 may not be true. There is also another, more complicated theory to explain this action. Both these ideas are discussed by Dr Hans Nieper of Hanover in his articles on New Approaches to Cancer Therapy. (M. Kochi et al. *Cancer Treatment*, Rep. 64:21, 1980.)

But why probe the difficult biochemical principles when results speak for themselves? We are dealing with natural substances and if the remarkable people of Hunza aren't evidence enough, there are literally thousands of cancer patients in the USA and other parts of the world who already know from personal experience that Vitamin B-17 in conjunction with other dietary measures has an anti-cancer action.

The Laetrile (B-17) Controversy

For more than two decades now opposing factions in the USA have been arguing the pros and cons of laetrile as a cancer therapy. Laetrile is a medicinal extract of B-17 derived from apricot kernels. Amygdalin is another name for laetrile.

The United States Federal Drug Administration (FDA), which screens all medicines before allowing them to be prescribed to the public, has continually insisted that laetrile must not be used for cancer treatment. Only the determination of a small but courageous lobby of doctors and patients has prevented the complete suppression of B-17 in the United States.

The FDA objection to the use of B-17 as an anti-cancer agent is that it gives false hope to patients. Certainly doctors using B-17 to treat their patients have risked being struck off the medical register.

Largely due to public pressure, there are today 27 States where B-17 is allowed for cancer treatment providing the doctor applying for supplies gives his written assurance that he is only going to give it to a patient who is dying.

And all this official caution focused on a non-toxic food factor which can both protect and influence the course of cancer!

The political suppression of Amygdalin/Laetrile/B-17 in the USA has been well documented. (*World Without Cancer* by G. Edward Griffin.) FDA sponsored 'trials' of this vitamin have also been widely publicised in an attempt to dissuade people from asking for it.

Experts in the field of nutritional therapy insist that the testing of laetrile by the National Cancer Institute was deliberately biased.

Cancer patients invited to take part in the clinical trials were practically moribund. There were no controls. They were also made aware that the doctors administering their doses of laetrile had no faith in the product. Only a casual attempt was made to incorporate into the 'trials' the diet and other vitamins essential for a good response. It is also alleged that the supplies of Vitamin B-17 used were not sufficiently fresh or properly stabilised.

Today, after nearly 20 years of argument, most people in the States who want B-17 treatment for cancer have to cross the Mexican border to one or other of the excellent natural therapy clinics which are forced to operate outside the jurisdiction of the FDA.

The Del Mar Clinic, Tihuana, Mexico

Dr Ernesto Contreras, the doctor in charge of the Del Mar Clinic has for more than ten years been giving cancer patients B-17 in conjunction with a special diet and other vitamin supplements. Considering that most of his patients are usually suffering advanced cancer which has already been treated by orthodox interventions, the results achieved by Contreras and his medical colleagues is astonishing.

Since the clinic opened, well over 30,000 people have been treated there with Vitamin B-17 and diet. None has suffered any toxic effects and 45 per cent were able to enjoy an improved quality of life even though the disease process had progressed too far to save them.

Amygdalin (also a medicinal derivative of B-17) as an anti-tumour agent has additional advantages. It relieves pain and/or fetor when these are present.

Dr Contreras has treated 257 patients with inoperable lung cancer. These patients were not expected to survive for more than six months but with non-toxic treatment lived on with a good quality of life for 14 months. Five per cent of these patients made a complete recovery.

At the Del Mar Clinic, cancer patients are involved in a daily programme of wholistic therapies aimed at cleansing the system of toxins and restoring internal conditions which enhance the body's natural healing abilities.

Contreras and his medical team are supported in their work by two psychologists and two spiritual healers. Patients who are terminally ill when they arrive, are surrounded by an atmosphere of love, honesty about their condition and treatment, and understanding of their fears and feelings of helplessness. The positive emotional support offered is in itself a healing factor.

There are numerous other clinics in Mexico and elsewhere offering cancer patients non-toxic treatments which include amygdalin. However, not all provide the integrated 'total person' approach which Dr Contreras was among the first to pioneer.

At his Silbersee Clinic in Hanover, West Germany, Dr Hans Nieper combines orthodox and non-toxic cancer regimes, often with dramatic results, but the emphasis is on 'treating the symptoms' of cancer.

In Bavaria there's the Ringberg Clinic, founded by Dr Joseph Issels; in Holland the Moerman Clinic also working along naturopathic lines; in Jamaica the Fairfield Clinic, similar to the Gerson Clinic in Mexico, giving patients juice diets and vitamin therapy. But apart from the Del Mar, the first to offer the entire range of wholistic therapies is the Bristol Centre in the UK.

Unfortunately treatment at private cancer clinics is costly. However, quite recently the medical insurance agency BUPA reimbursed a large percentage of the expenses incurred by one member who went to Mexico for treatment, and certainly Bristol has already set up bursaries to defray the cost of treatment for less affluent patients – at least until such time as this centre is recognised by the NHS.

The Vitamin C Controversy

Irwin Stone, author of *The Healing Factor* and one of the world's principle researchers into the benefits of Vitamin C, told the following story when lecturing to a Cancer Convention in Los Angeles in 1973.

'A dog in the last stages of distemper was taken to a veterinary hospital. The animal was comatose and hadn't eaten for a week. The vet injected the dog with 12 grammes of sodium ascorbate (Vitamin C) and put him in a pen. He then went into the hospital kitchen and opened a can of dog food. When he returned, the dog was jumping around the enclosure, and when given the food, gobbled it voraciously. In the short interval since the injection, its temperature had returned to normal and after a few more daily shots of Vitamin C (in megadoses) it was sent home cured.'

Adele Davis, the American nutritionist, also used megadoses of Vitamin C on her children when they suffered any of the usual childhood infections, well aware of this vitamin's remarkable antibiotic properties. In this way she transformed measles and mumps into one-day illnesses!

Dr Frederick Klenner was another pioneer enthusiast for the efficacy of Vitamin C in large dosage and frequently administered it intravenously in doses of two to four grammes throughout the day to desperately-ill patients who responded dramatically.

Drs Linus Pauling and Albert Szent-Gyorgyi received Nobel Prizes for their scientific work with Vitamin C, and at the Vale of Leven Hospital in Scotland, Dr Ewan Cameron conducted a trial with terminally-ill cancer patients. Those given *megadoses* of ascorbic acid gained extensive remissions. A few survived to regain their health. (Proceedings of the National Academy of Sciences, 1978.)

All this provocative research – a mere snippet of what has been recorded throughout the last twenty years – is still largely ignored by the medical establishment, who prefer to prescribe chemical drugs rather than a natural and inexpensive vitamin with no toxic side-effects.

Much of the criticism levelled at Vitamin C is due to giving it in doses other than *large amounts*. It is the *megadoses* which prove the remarkable healing properties of ascorbic acid, as illustrated in the story of Maurice Burke, who in desperation, but with excellent serendipity, persuaded his doctors to give him Vitamin C for terminal cancer.

Towards the end of 1975 Burke noticed a small lump on the side of his neck. Because his work as an industrial engineer frequently took him abroad, he thought he'd picked up an infection in one of the South American countries he'd recently visited.

Back home in Canada he was examined by doctors at the Ottawa Hospital for Tropical Diseases but given a clean bill of health.

By 1978 Burke and his wife had gone to live in Switzerland. Now the lump in his neck had become so large it was causing a certain amount of embarrassment, so Burke went to the Berne hospital for an exploratory operation.

When he came round from the anaesthetic Maurice Burke could scarcely speak. His surgeon told him that they'd removed a large carcinoma of the left neck triangle which involved the jugular vein and the recurrent nerve. It was the severance of this nerve which had reduced Burke's voice to a whisper.

Maurice Burke was given a course of chemotherapy. This made him so ill he soon refused to continue it. So he was given a new and expensive cancer treatment involving injections of Interferon. Three months later the growth in his neck had recurred.

Once more he was admitted to hospital where he was given cobalt therapy to reduce the swelling as a preliminary to another operation. He became desperate.

'I felt I would die shortly. I sent for my sons in Canada to visit me and when, after a short visit, they left to go home, I was certain I'd never see them again.'

An aggressive course of radiotherapy to his neck was started. Over five weeks Burke had 5000 rems of radiation which was the maximum dose allowed. He suffered skin burns, loss of his hair and the salivary glands on the left side of his mouth ceased to function. He also got thrombo-phlebitis in his left leg, a known complication of excessive radiotherapy.

'By then I was a complete wreck,' Maurice recalled. 'I could only talk in a whisper, I couldn't climb stairs without gasping for breath. All I had to look forward to was another operation which by all accounts would be particularly disfiguring.

'Only then did it occur to me that I ought to make the effort to take some responsibility for my own life and think seriously about finding another solution to my cancer.'

Reading everything he could find on unorthodox cancer treatments, Burke soon found himself immersed in a vast amount of written material. Eventually he came across an article 'Vitamin C and Cancer' by Dominic Bosco in the magazine *Prevention*. What he read convinced him that if he could persuade his local GP to co-operate, he might still have a fighting chance.

Burke was fortunate. His doctor arranged for him to have a daily infusion of 20 gm of Vitamin C. The small hospital in Burke's hometown of Gstaad had to send away for this amount which was more than they normally used in a whole year.

Each day for four days Maurice Burke lay on a hospital bed with an intravenous drip of Vitamin C in his arm. Nothing happened until the fifth day when Burke suddenly realised he was feeling better.

'For the first time in months it felt good to be alive,' he recalled.

After nine days the intravenous treatment was stopped because Burke's arm had become too sore. Instead he substituted a daily oral amount of 16 grammes of Vitamin C divided into four doses. He also researched the value of other vitamins which might stimulate his recovery and began to take large amounts of Vitamin A, Vitamin E and the mineral Selenium.

Six weeks later Burke's neck suddenly swelled alarmingly, filling the whole area of his left neck from jaw to collarbone. His immediate reaction was to believe the vitamin therapy had failed, but as he continued to feel perfectly well, he persevered with the treatment.

Three weeks later the swelling began to subside. Two months later it had completely disappeared. So had the thrombosis in his leg.

In 1980 orthodox tests showed that Maurice Burke no longer had any trace of cancer. Today he is well and living in Warwickshire.

Sceptics will argue that Maurice Burke was an example of 'spontaneous remission'; or that the original diagnosis was wrong. Yet here is an example of someone who is living proof of the connection between cancer and the nutrients in the food we eat, a connection demonstrated even more clearly by Dr Max Gerson, the New York Physician who for more than 30 years successfully treated patients with juice diets.

Dr Max Gerson

An emigré to the United States from Germany, in the early 1930s until his death in 1959 at the age of 80 Max Gerson practised medicine in New York, gaining a reputation as a doctor who could successfully treat chronic degenerative diseases – including cancer – with a special diet. This was based on his firm belief (and clinical observations) that once the human body was given the right kind of nutritional help it was capable of cleansing the system of disease.

The Gerson programme was salt-free and based on fresh-pressed raw fruit and vegetable juices and the juice of fresh liver.

To stimulate the liver in its work of cleansing toxins out of the body, the patient also took frequent coffee enemas (see page 138).

In 1946 Gerson was called before a Senate Subcommittee

to describe his work with cancer patients. The senators were so impressed by what they heard that they promised to recommend large sums of government money for thorough research into Gerson's methods. Before these recommendations could go forward for approval the Subcommittee hearing had to be reviewed by the medical authorities of the day.

Dr Max Gerson was subsequently branded as a quack and a fraud. The medical authorities which demanded that all orthodox therapies be subjected to stringent scientific scrutiny denied Gerson's work the same attention despite the many people who came forward to testify that his nutritional therapy had saved their lives when 'scientifically tested' treatments had failed.

Max Gerson's book *A Cancer Therapy: Results of Fifty Cases* was published after his death. It contains the meticulously documented medical case histories of 50 cancer patients each one diagnosed and treated by orthodox cancer specialists before turning to Dr Gerson for help. Most of these people were ultimately restored to health.

Today at La Gloria Clinic (obliged, like most of the others offering nutritional cancer therapy, to operate across the California border in Mexico) Max Gerson's daughter and a team of medical specialists continue to use the therapies devised by the man Albert Schweitzer called 'a genius who walked amongst us'.

There are at least 80 non-toxic therapy measures designed to control cancer which have been extensively and effectively used considering that in most cases patients only turn to this kind of help when all else fails.

Some gentle therapies favour herbs. Others place the emphasis on enzymes or fruit juice fasts or buckwheat grass or inducing fever in the patient to stimulate auto-immune responses. But in all of them there is always a consistent theme.

The treatment must cleanse toxic substances from the patient's body and stimulate the natural functioning of the immune system.

The roll-call of eminent non-toxic practitioners is long and impressive. Names such as William Kelley, Paavo Airola, Harry Hoxey, Irwin Stone, Dean Burke, John Richardson, Oscar Todd, Contreras and Gerson; biochemists like the Krebses and Linus Pauling and many more. All these highly trained people have published results of their work with cancer patients, and it seems inconceivable that there can possibly be any further intelligent argument about whether or not nutritional factors have a part to play in cancer control.

When we talk of health, there is nothing that can be usefully added to pure air, pure water, wholesome food and harmonious living to improve them. The Hunzakuts are a living example of that.

When it comes to cancer, the knowledge that thousands of patients have actually eaten their way to recovery should finally dispel the aura of fear which surrounds this illness called cancer.

6 THE BRISTOL DIET

This is the first of three chapters which describe in detail the self-help programmes offered to patients attending the Bristol Cancer Help Centre. They are designed by Dr Alec Forbes and based on methods which have been widely and effectively used by him and other reliable practitioners.

These programmes for The Diet, Metabolic Therapy, Self-healing, Psychotherapy and Healing are explained separately but always used together. This is the total therapy approach for cancer control. But it should always be remembered that no two cancer patients respond in the same way so the therapies are often adapted to suit individual needs, according to the advice of the therapists in charge.

Getting Started

Newcomers to the BCHC sometimes find the idea of having to abandon many of their old eating habits and get used to a diet which may at first seem unpalatable, a daunting prospect. Therapists at the centre are well aware of this, and will go to great lengths to explain exactly what the diet part of the wholistic programme is intended to achieve, how it is carefully designed to cleanse toxins out of the body whilst at the same time stimulate the patient's natural recuperative powers.

Despite this encouragement, there are always some patients who decide that the effort and sacrifices involved are just not worthwhile. Which is why the BCHC insists that before people book in to attend the clinics, they first write for the specially-prepared kit of recorded cassettes and leaflets. In this way they can decide beforehand whether or not they are capable of making the necessary dietary changes.

Then again, some patients visiting the centre have already started on the diet and are already feeling the benefits, which is a fine first step towards an appreciation of what self-help therapies are all about.

The Diet Excludes Meat

The possibility that a meatless meal can be both appetising and nourishing often surprises people, especially if they also believe that 'wholefood' and vegetarianism constitute examples of 'cranky eating'. Yet prior to the last war, the normal diet was nothing else but 'wholefood' – that is food produced by organic cultivation methods and reaching the consumer with the minimum of refining and processing.

Nor is meat the only reliable source of protein. Fish, eggs and dairy products are, of course, high-protein foods, but none of these (except yoghurt) are included in the anti-cancer diet, which is deliberately low in protein. But first a word about normal protein requirements.

The cancer-free Hunzakuts (Chapter 5) eat less than half the protein contained in the average western diet and live a lot longer than the average western citizen. Their diet is derived from cereals, vegetables, beans and, of course, those delicious little apricots with their nitriloside-rich kernels.

In the last decade nutritionists have revised their assessment of how much daily protein is needed to maintain health. Once this was thought to be in excess of 70 grammes daily. Now it is believed that optimum health can be easily maintained on much less; a daily intake of 56 protein grammes for men and 46 for women. (American Academy of Sciences, 1974.)

However the diet designed at Bristol is even lower in protein content because it is going to provide much more than just straightforward nourishment. The diet must also create the best possible internal conditions for tumour destruction, and this is best achieved by eating fresh foods rich in organic enzymes and containing only enough protein to stimulate the pancreas to produce the enzymes particularly associated with dissolving the protein covering on cancer cells which enables them to evade the body's natural defences against disease.

If meat or any other high-protein foods were included in the diet, this would divert pancreatic enzymes from tumour destruction to the work of digesting, thereby defeating the whole object of the exercise.

So the Bristol diet is derived from fresh vegetables, fruit, wholegrain cereals, and sprouted beans and seeds, all carefully combined to ensure that the patient gets a nutritionally balanced diet. But having once accepted a diet without meat, the new patient now has to face another dietary challenge.

At least 70 per cent of the diet is composed of raw food – for excellent reasons.

It is common knowledge that cooking destroys some of the vitamin content of foodstuffs. Less well-known is the fact that heat destroys *all the enzymes*. And enzymes, as already explained, are needed in tremendous quantities. These are the live elements in fresh, uncooked vegetables.

Grated raw vegetables and salads (juiced when the patient has difficulty swallowing) form the first and most important part of every meal. Then, if the person still feels hungry, the diet allows lentil and vegetable soups, jacket potatoes, wholemeal bread, and a variety of other wholesome foods. It may seem a spartan diet until you begin to appreciate how every meal is cleansing your system and stimulating the internal chemistry which seeks to eliminate cancer. That is why you need raw, fresh and wholesome foods, and anything that impedes this objective should be strictly avoided.

Please – No Junk Food!

In the western world, during the course of a single year, each person eats about half a ton of food. Much of this is riddled with chemicals. There are some 3000 additives in the food which appears on supermarket shelves, and although a quick look at the labelling will reveal that the contents contain 'permitted' artificial preservatives or colouring etc., the 1965 government committee formed to monitor the food industry's alliance with the chemical industry can offer no guarantees concerning the absolute safety of these artificial ingredients.

This means that if one food contains a small amount of an additive considered 'safe', no one knows how it might react in the human body with other chemical food additives to form a substance far from safe. Nor have tests been done to find out what might happen if someone hooked on, say, instant desserts, eats large amounts of this 'food' in one day.

As for the possible long-term accumulative effects of food additives, nobody can predict the outcome of this. What is predicted is that over the next decade the food industry will be increasing chemical additives in foods. And already there is growing evidence that this is having a positively harmful effect on some people.

For instance, tartrazine, the yellow dye put into cakes, cheese, medicines, sweets and many other foods, is strongly suspected of causing hyperactivity in some children and allergies in some adults, particularly those intolerant to aspirin.

Research in the USA now suggests children should avoid artificial colouring altogether. Maybe we all should, if we want to live to a healthy old age. It seems that the adulteration of the food we eat has now gone beyond the control of the Food Standards Committee. It is therefore up to the individual, who is well informed about the dangers of food additives, agricultural pesticides and so forth, to exercise common sense in order to protect his own interests.

As for the cancer patient, you have to make doubly sure that what you eat is unadulterated and wholesome. Which may well mean that a lot of things you are used to eating will have to go: tinned foods (those loaded with sugar and salt), carbonated drinks, fish-fingers, instant snacks, frozen chips, instant soups and desserts, pickles, bottled sauces, crisps, biscuits, and anything else that comes under the heading of 'junk' (de-natured) food.

Know *what* you should be eating, *why* you are eating it, and *how* it is improving your health. Then you can't go far wrong.

Alcohol, Coffee & Tea

These are also omitted from the anti-cancer diet because they are artificial stimulants which put an extra strain on the liver. And in all patients, liver-function is impaired. Also, the caffeine in tea and coffee inhibits the production of those important pancreatic enzymes. Another good reason to cut coffee out of the diet is because the solvent called trichlorethylene used in the manufacture of decaffeinated ground and instant coffee, accumulates in the body over long periods and is a chemical known to cause cancer in laboratory mice.

However, for those of you who enjoy it, a little alcohol daily is allowed for medicinal reasons! But not much. Two medium glasses of good white wine or two tots of spirit can be drunk, because it has been found that this encourages the secretion of prostaglandin E1 – another front-line player in the body's defence-league against disease.

Salt is Omitted from the Diet

Because it is linked with high blood pressure and the increasing incidence of heart attacks, for some time now doctors have been advising people to cut down on salt. Adding salt to food – as adding sugar to food – is unnecessary, since both occur naturally. The trouble is that the food industry adds so much salt to processed foodstuffs that people have got into the habit of eating about ten times more than they actually need.

So adapting to a salt-free diet requires patience. Start by cooking without salt and then adding a little at the table. Gradually cut this down and soon you will find that as the natural food flavours re-educate your taste-buds, going without salt altogether will be no hardship.

As an added incentive to giving up salt, you should know that in the body it is salt which inhibits cell life and potassium which enhances it. Ideally there should be a balance between potassium in the cells and sodium (salt) outside. When this balance is destroyed by eating too much salt, this reverses the situation and loss of potassium from the cells exposes them to disease.

Eat Food That is Organically Grown

Certainly with current agricultural policies, this isn't always easy to do, especially for those who live in urban areas without gardens. However, since this book was first published and the needs of cancer patients are more properly understood, several organisations have come forward to offer help with locating sources of organically-grown vegetables – particularly carrots.

These associations are listed on page 176 at the back of this book.

Sprouting Seeds & Grains

The way to get a constant supply of home-grown, high quality vitamin and enzyme rich vegetable matter is to grow beansprouts in the airing cupboard.

You can buy specially stacked plastic trays to sprout grains and seeds but there is an equally efficient method. In a large, clean glass jar, put a handful of seeds (see list below) and tie a square of porous cloth over the opening. (A piece of nylon stocking would do.) Pour in warm water to cover the seeds and soak for a few hours. Then drain off the water, turn the jar on its side and shake the seeds along its length. Leave the jar in a warm, dark place (which is why the airing-cupboard is suggested) and once or twice a day repeat the rinsing.

Depending upon the type of seed, germination occurs within three to five days. When sprouts appear, bring the jar into the light. Keep up the watering routine and when the sprouts have grown to about an inch, use them in salads – or for making wholewheat sandwiches. They are crunchy, deliciously flavoured and ORGANICALLY GROWN by you in a matter of days!

SUITABLE BEANS, SEEDS AND GRAINS FOR SPROUTING

Ask for them in your local wholefood shop. The asterisked varieties are rich in B-17.

Mung beans*	Alfalfa*	Buckwheat*
Lentils*	Aduki beans	Chickpeas
Soy beans	Sunflower seeds	Sesame seeds

Occasionally, a few seeds in a batch do not germinate. Remove these before making salads.

All beansprouts are rich in Vitamins A, B-2, C and E. Also potassium. Above all they provide an excellent source of those important anti-cancer enzymes.

The beansprouts which provide a rich natural source of Vitamin B-17 also contribute to another aspect of tumour destruction. The protein-digesting enzymes de-shield the tumour and the active anti-cancer constituents of B-17, which is concentrated into Laetrile, destroy the malignant cells. (This process is explained in Chapter 5.)

So the four principles of the anti-cancer diet are:

Fresh vegetables, fruits, cereals, pulse and juices
No meat or dairy products (at least to begin with)
No junk foods
70% raw food.

This is the basis for the Bristol Diet. It simultaneously nourishes the patient's system as it causes tumour destruction and is not a 'swings and roundabouts' treatment which attacks the cancer at the expense of the immune system.

Obviously individuals have different responses to the diet. Some begin to feel an improvement in a week or so, others – and especially those who find it difficult to abandon lifelong eating habits – may take longer. But the proven fact is that everybody who sticks to the diet benefits.

Given to someone just recovering from a bad attack of influenza – or a stay in hospital – the Bristol Diet would be a wonderful way to hasten convalescence. But the health of the cancer patient has been seriously undermined over a long period. There's a considerable backlog of nutritional repair work to be done. This is why Vitamin supplements are added to the daily menu to give an additional boost to the diet's overall effectiveness.

By the time they arrive at the BCHC, some patients are already very ill. Their appetites are poor and the prospect of having to eat large helpings of raw vegetables and salads fills them with dismay. Patients with tumours in the throat, stomach or bowels will already have serious vitamin deficiencies, as cancer leeches vitamins and minerals from whatever is eaten to sustain its own peculiar development. So someone with advanced disease is without the nutritional building blocks necessary to repair and activate the very defence mechanisms which destroy malignant tumours. In these cases, the diet (juiced if necessary) is supplemented by a range of vitamin and mineral tablets.

What are Vitamins?

These are food factors necessary for correct metabolism. (Metabolism is the way the body absorbs and converts food and oxygen into growth and energy.)

The body can't manufacture vitamins. These always come from the food we eat. Diets which lack one or more of the essential vitamins can eventually cause a variety of serious ailments. Some growing children, deprived of Vitamin D, suffer from rickets or poor bone formation. In the Third World, where there is a diet-deficiency of Vitamin A, blindness can result. These are just two examples of what might happen when diets are deficient in one or more vitamins. And replacing those lost vitamins is also the remedy.

But normally a well-balanced diet provides all the vitamins essential for health. Vitamin supplements given to cancer patients are given in doses far larger than those usually recommended, because their systems are already seriously depleted in vitamins and minerals. There is a lot of 'repair work' to be done.

Vitamin Supplements Taken with the Bristol Diet

If the patient is having the full range of substances which comprise the Metabolic Therapy programme, some or all of the following vitamins will be included in it.

If the patient chooses to omit the more strenuous Metabolic Therapy regime, designed to speed up tumour destruction, then the diet with vitamin supplements and the mind-over-matter exercises explained in Chapter 9 will achieve the same results, but perhaps over a longer period of time.

These, then, are the vitamins which play a vital role in the anti-cancer diet.

VITAMIN A

This supplement comes from fresh-pressed carrot juice (carotene) which the patient makes with the use of an electrical juice extractor. However, so that Vitamin A is not stored in the liver but made to circulate in the system, carrot juice is emulsified with a teaspoonful of cold-pressed oil, whisked for not less than one minute in a liquidiser.

It is Vitamin A flushed to the site of the tumours which enhances the action of nitrilosides in the diet – those food factors known as Vitamin B-17, or as chemical derivatives called Amygdalin or Laetrile.

Vitamin A plays a crucial role in helping to resist cancer. All patients have low blood levels of this vitamin, which the immune system needs in large quantities when subjected to severe physical stresses resulting from chronic ill-health and/or surgery.

Research into the relationship between Vitamin A and cancer goes back to 1942, when at the University of Texas it was found that in animal cancer experiments, those animals given Vitamin A before radiation treatment reduced the amount of radiation required to control the tumour by 25 per cent.

Since then, numerous studies definitely show that a deficiency in Vitamin A contributes to the development of malignancies.

Vitamin A is one of the most important aids to the body's defensive system in the fight to control (and prevent) cancer.

Dosage is about $1\frac{1}{2}$ pints (900 mls) spread over the day.

VITAMIN B

This is contained in brewer's yeast (powder or tablet form) and in wholewheat bread, brown rice and yoghurt, all of which are allowed in the diet and feature in the recipes on pages 110-124.

However, for those who dislike the taste of brewer's yeast sprinkled into soups or over stews, tablets can be taken instead with meals. Dosage is given on the bottle.

VITAMIN C

This vitamin (ascorbic acid) reinforces the action of Vitamin A and is probably the most potent anti-toxin known when taken in *large doses*. Then Vitamin C inhibits an enzyme called hyaluronidase, found in cancerous tissues.

It has been found in clinical application that the sicker the person is, the greater his digestive tolerance to Vitamin C. A patient with a viral pneumonia can tolerate in excess of 200 grammes! But these large doses are usually given intravenously, so none of the effect is lost in the digestive tract.

As well as strengthening connective tissues (collagen) and being the anti-stress vitamin, Vitamin C also has analgesic properties. Above all, this vitamin stimulates the production of the T-lymphocytes, the potent forces in the bloodstream associated with the destruction of infection and chronic disease.

The minimum dosage daily advised is 6 grammes. This can be in tablet form, each tablet containing 500 mlgs, or in powdered form dissolved in water.

VITAMIN E

Cancer cells don't like oxygen! This vitamin increases the oxygenation of the cells and – like Vitamin C – inhibits the activity of the enzyme involved in cancer-cell growth.

However, this supplement is not recommended for patients with hormone-related cancer ie: of the breast and female reproductive organs. (This reservation does not apply to cancer of the prostate.)

The daily dose is 100 i.u. three times daily with meals for seven days; then twice this amount for the next week; after that, take 400 i.u. of Vitamin E twice every day as a maintenance dose.

MINERAL SUPPLEMENTS

One important part of the Bristol diet is to adjust the so-called 'mineral carriers'. These are compounds in the food we eat which carry magnesium, potassium, calcium and zinc to the different sites of the cells.

Potassium and magnesium activate energy-rich phosphates which are in the forefront of the body's immune defence system. Iron orotate also strengthens this defence system. But these minerals are (or should be) in the food we eat, derived from healthy soil which has not had the mineral content depleted by the use of artificial cultivation methods.

If you think of the body as a kind of human battery, it is minerals which charge the cellular structure to fight malignant diseases. And cancer patients are almost always seriously deficient in five most important minerals; potassium, magnesium, selenium, zinc and calcium.

SELENIUM

Selenium is an interesting anti-oxidant. Too much is a positive health hazard. So is none at all!

Studies around the world have shown that where the mineral selenium is naturally present in the soil, cancer is never a problem. In the UK there is an area of Norfolk where the soil is rich in this mineral and the incidence of cancer there is below the average for the country as a whole.

This observation was confirmed by a survey done by the magazine *Prevention* in 1973, when the blood of 1000 people who had cancer was tested for its selenium content.

Compared with people who were healthy, it was shown that cancer patients were seriously lacking in this mineral.

Many other laboratory tests indicate that selenium is a necessary diet supplement for cancer patients. Experiments on laboratory mice given selenium showed that they produced a third more anti-bodies than mice on a diet without it, thus demonstrating the importance of this mineral in the body's defence mechanisms against disease.

Although the amount needed is minute, the anti-oxidant property of selenium has been shown to have significant results in experiments done on human cancer patients.

Researchers at the Cleveland Clinic Foundation in the USA examined human blood cells taken from volunteer donors and observed microscopic chromosomal breaks in their cancer cells. They found that adding a chemical anti-oxidant prompted faulty cells to repair themselves. Adding Vitamin C also reinforced this effect, but when the scientists added the mineral selenium, cell damage was reduced by a spectacular 41 per cent.

This experiment would seem to confirm the use of anti-oxidants as a protection against chromosomal damage closely related to two aspects of human frailty: ageing and cancer.

Best sources of selenium are brewer's yeast, wholewheat, asparagus, mushrooms (allowed on diet), liver and seafoods (which are not).

Supplement dosage is one 200 mcg tablet daily.

MAGNESIUM

As with selenium, when levels of magnesium in the soil are high, the incidence of cancer is lower than average.

The role of magnesium is crucial to the proper functioning of the living cell, and it has been found that when the cell's supply of magnesium becomes drastically reduced, its metabolic functions start to limp and lag.

'Magnesium,' Dr Harry Rubin, Professor of Molecular

Biology at the University of California, once said, 'is the only substance that has an effect on every pathway to the cell. It is the universal controller of all cell life and cancer, as we should never forget, is primarily a cellular disturbance.' That is why adequate magnesium in the anti-cancer diet is imperative.

Magnesium should be present in sufficient amounts in the food we eat. Unfortunately today this is often not the case because of food processing. Wheat, one rich source of magnesium, loses 85 per cent of its magnesium content when bleached into white flour. The same loss happens when fresh vegetables are canned and when cow's milk is used instead of mother's milk to feed babies.

It is lack of magnesium in the soil which deprives vegetables of flavour. It is the indiscriminate use of artificial fertilisers and pesticides which destroys the magnesium (and other minerals) in healthy soil.

Because magnesium and calcium work in tandem in the body, supplements of magnesium are given together with calcium in tablets called Dolomite. The dosage is given on the bottle. Otherwise, foods rich in magnesium include nuts, seeds, molasses, bananas, etc., when the magnesium/calcium balance is naturally present.

ZINC

Try to think of the cells in the body as functioning along the lines of a battery. Then it is minerals like potassium and magnesium which charge the human battery, activating the vital enzymes (including pancreatic enzymes) which protect cells against malignancy.

Zinc deficiency slows down the healing of wounds, stunts the growth of sex organs, reduces the sense of smell, and contributes to ulcers and prostate problems. It can even lead to male impotency.

Zinc may also have something to do with intelligence,

since people with high IQs have been shown to have consistently higher levels of this mineral in their systems.

Loss of zinc from soil and from our food is due to the same sad story. Artificial methods of cultivation and food processing over the last three decades have meant that people have not been getting enough zinc in their diets. Alcohol and too much refined sugar also leeches this important mineral from body tissues.

The best way to increase zinc intake is to eat more herrings, seafood, meat, eggs, and wheatgerm. But on the Bristol diet only wheatgerm is allowed. So zinc supplements are necessary in daily doses of at least 15 mgs, probably more, but this would depend upon individual needs assessed by wholeblood analysis.

POTASSIUM

In the healthy body potassium remains largely in the cells and sodium in the surrounding tissue fluids. Both play a vital part in controlling the cellular passage of nutrients and other essential substances. When the potassium content of the cells decreases because the diet lacks sufficient of this mineral, sodium can pass into the depleted cells. Then tissues become waterlogged and common results are high blood pressure and dropsy.

Chronic stress also causes the cells to lose potassium and store salt, and because stress is invariably a problem with cancer patients, they are almost always suffering from potassium deficiency. That is why the Bristol diet is salt-free and potassium-rich, and why lack of potassium in the average diet is due to dependency on processed food.

For instance, a 3½ oz (90 gm) helping of *fresh* garden peas contains 316 mg of potassium but only 2 mgs of mineral salt. When this same quantity of peas is canned for the supermarket shelf, it contains a massive 236 mgs of salt but only 96 mgs of potassium. The heat, the added sugar and other chemicals involved wreck the natural balance between sodium (salt) and potassium.

Potassium supplements are given in the form of 200 mgs daily in a tablet called Potassium Orotate. This dose may be increased if the patient is suffering from vomiting or diarrhoea, as both these symptoms drive potassium from the system.

These are five mineral supplements which accompany the anti-cancer diet. There are others which could be usefully taken, such as iodine in the form of Kelp tablets, and tablets which combine potassium and Vitamin C. Then it's just a question of putting aside all other considerations and for two or three months concentrating on the daily programme of gentle therapies.

Try to Obtain Your Doctor's Co-operation

Patients who follow the wholistic programme are advised to inform their doctors so as to keep the relationship on the best possible footing. And since the BCHC first opened, a lot more physicians are aware of these therapies and what can (and has) been achieved by using them.

Your doctor may be only too willing to prescribe some, if not all, of the vitamins and mineral supplements. On the other hand, if he declines to do so, don't be discouraged. Work hard on the anti-cancer diet, and once your health improves you can then ask again for his help in the expectation that when your doctor sees the improvement he will be only too glad to assist you maintain it in any way he can.

Cancer is a Systemic Disease

Those who believe that cancer is the result of a gradual

breakdown of body defences also believe the anti-cancer diet, the vitamin and mineral supplements, and (if chosen) the Metabolic Therapy Programme can arrest tumour growth and then slowly reverse the disease process.

When this occurs, the revitalised immune system doesn't just throw out cancer and leave any other unhealthy condition which may be present. Treating the whole system with nutrition means that it is the whole system that ultimately benefits.

However, patients who have had one 'attack' of cancer should always watch their diet, just as a diabetic has to maintain health by observing certain nutritional rules.

At the Bristol Centre, during its early days, there was a lady schoolteacher who went to learn the therapy measures and derived such benefits from them that she joined the staff as a voluntary counsellor.

She had been operated on for breast cancer and not long afterwards suffered painful 'secondary' growths on the site of the mastectomy.

Her consultant wanted to operate again, but instead she chose to follow the Bristol programme. The new cancer growths disappeared.

'I then felt so much better, I decided it would be safe to relax the diet programme and start to have more of the foods I was used to eating. But within two weeks, back had come my painful little lumps! So back I went onto the 70 per cent raw food diet and away went the lumps.

'I then deliberately stopped the diet to make sure that this was really the cause of my relapse. Sure enough, the 'secondaries' returned. This proved to me beyond all doubt that my system needed all the nutrients in the diet not just some of the time but all of the time. It was a salutary lesson!'

Fresh is Best

Kirlian photography is able to demonstrate that all living

organisms are surrounded by an electro-magnetic energy field.

The 'aura' surrounding a leaf can be captured on film. When a piece is cut away, the energy field which appears on the film is as if the leaf was still intact! But thereafter this 'aura' slowly fades.

Similarly, live foods, grown by natural cultivation methods, sustain a high life-force field for quite a while after they have been picked, but as freshness deteriorates, their energy decreases.

Kirlian photography has also been used to film the energy field around people. In this way it has been possible to compare the integrated 'aura' of a healthy person with the broken energy field around somebody who is sick.

The cancer patient needs optimum enzyme and vitamin nourishment from the raw food diet, so should try to prepare and eat food that is extremely fresh – whenever possible, vegetables that have also been organically cultivated.

The life-force in pure, live, raw food nourishes the life-force of the body.

Prepare with Love – Eat With a Prayer

Vegetables cultivated by organic means are sometimes difficult to obtain. But in the last two years, as the needs of cancer patients on special diets have become more widely recognised, an increasing number of market-gardeners are turning to organic cultivation.

However, it has to be said that some 'health food' shops are more interested in profits than in providing genuinely organic produce. So it's up to the cancer patient to know exactly what he wants and then set out to get it from reliable sources.

Some patients will have good neighbours willing to part with garden produce. Then again, when all else fails, don't forget the super-nourishment of home-grown beansprouts.

If you have to use vegetables of 'doubtful' origin, wash them thoroughly and then 'prepare with love and eat with a prayer'.

There was much wisdom in the old practice of saying 'grace' before meals. This act of blessing calms the nervous system and 'tunes' the appetite, so the maximum goodness can be absorbed from what is eaten.

What About Exercise?

Even cancer patients who feel quite ill should make an effort to do some form of daily exercise – even if it is only stretching exercises in the living-room. A walk in the fresh air would be better. Exercise is important.

In 1977 at a research institute in Japan, laboratory mice were given benzidine which is a powerful carcinogen. Then one group of mice were put in a cage with an exercise wheel. The other group were left without one.

In the group that exercised, 63 per cent developed cancer. In the group which did not exercise, the incidence was 93 per cent.

Of course you are no mouse! But do try and make time during the day for some form of physical exercise to stimulate circulation and breathing and generally tone up the system.

Healthy Surroundings

Try to cut down on all those sprays, detergents and other household substances which everyone has become used to having about the home. Almost all of them contain substances which can – over time – damage your health.

If a bunch of nettles keeps flies out, forget about fly sprays. Do without those aerosol air fresheners, deodorant sprays in the bathroom, hair lacquer – anything which means breathing in the contents of these modern dispensers.

If it's possible to make your home a no-smoking zone, so much the better. It's now known that even people who don't smoke but have to inhale the tobacco smoke of others, run as many risks from this carcinogen. However, if a ban on smoking causes too much family friction, at least invest in a negative ionizer. This little gadget will disperse 'fug' and freshen the air. It also has other benefits.

Research at Reading University's Department of Human Biology has established the health value of negative ionizers which produce what have been termed 'vitamins of the air'.

People who suffer from hay fever and migraine have had their symptoms relieved by these gadgets, and when coughs and colds are about, a negative ionizer in the room cuts down the risk of cross-infection within the family.

Juicing Machines

When Max Gerson devised his famous anti-cancer juice diets back in the 1950s, food-mixers lacked the sophistication of current models. Then Gerson insisted juices be extracted by hand-pressing, maintaining that valuable enzymes were destroyed by electric machines.

At Bristol they do not dispute the truth of this, but settle for a common-sense compromise. Patients use electric juicers and compensate for lost enzymes by taking enzyme supplements. (Bromelain/Papaya etc.)

There are numerous juicing machines on the market. Some are also food-processors. They can cost anything from around £50 to £200, but as the juicer (and liquidiser) is going to be in fairly constant use, patients are advised to look for one in the middle of this price range that will give reliable service.

The Maintenance Diet & Prevention

Taken on its own, the anti-cancer diet is particularly useful for cancer patients in the early stages of their illness. A more vigorous approach combines the diet with Metabolic Therapy, explained in Chapter 8. But it isn't only cancer patients who can benefit from the principles outlined in this book.

In the last three years there have been many instances of relatives who went on the diet to keep the cancer patient company and found that this greatly improved their health. Such complaints as piles, allergies, rheumatism, asthma and varicose veins are just some of the health problems that have cleared up as a result of re-organising usual eating habits.

Then again, people who want to safeguard against ill-health could do no better than start introducing raw food meals into their diets.

People who have had one 'attack' of cancer should always watch their diet, even when the disease has been controlled. Newfound and hard-won health is never again going to be content with anything but first-class nourishment.

Nature Knows Best

Learn to trust the marvellous self-healing properties of your own body. All you are required to do is give it the best possible conditions in which to do so. But remember: because cancer is the final symptom of a lengthy degenerative process, natural corrective measures are going to take time to produce results. Definite signs of improvement will be increased energy levels, a better appetite, and a general sense of well-being. By your own efforts you can turn *disease* into *ease*.

Once you realise the therapies are working, resist the temptation to slip back into old eating habits. Work at the programme one day at a time, bearing in mind that everything which improves basic health is another step in the right direction.

Exercise regularly, but whenever you feel tired, take a rest – preferably stretched out on the bed – or on the floor. (You'll be surprised how restful this can be!) Hot and cold showers tone up the circulation, and last, but by no means least, make sure to set aside regular intervals for the meditation exercises.

Think Positive!

Inevitably individual attitudes towards the future are of paramount importance. Also the attitude of the patient's close family. Regard cancer as an illness which *can* be overcome.

Certainly the struggle to regain your health will take determination and courage. If you have read thus far, you are probably the kind of person who will be able to harness these vital qualities.

7   RECIPES FOR RECOVERY

Nobody is suggesting that patients will be able to alter the habits of a lifetime overnight. Once you have a good idea of what the diet is designed to achieve, gradually ease yourself into the new daily programme, using the menus and recipes in this chapter to replace part and then all of the meals you've been accustomed to eating. And this will entail a certain amount of planning ahead.

If you haven't already got a liquidiser, you'll have to shop for this; also the juice-extractor if this is not included with the food-mixer.

Next you'll have to locate a regular supply of organically grown carrots and other vegetables. Carrot juice takes about 7 lbs of carrots daily. And since you'll be scrubbing these, not peeling them, get in some suitable bristle brushes and a long-handled bottle-brush for cleaning the bean-sprout jars (if you use this method) and also the thermos jug if you intend making your own yoghurt.

Treat yourself to some glass, stainless steel or iron cooking pots, and avoid using aluminium ones. Ask your local confectionery shop to sell you half a dozen of those big, wide-necked glass jars used for sweets. As well as using these to sprout seeds, they make excellent storage jars for mung beans, lentils, nuts, etc.

Organise a supply of bottled spring water, and if your mains supply of water is fluoridated, think very hard about fitting a filter gadget to the cold water tap. These cost around £50 and can be a saving if you are buying spring water over a long period. (Suppliers listed on page 176) But make sure from the manufacturer that the gadget really does filter out fluoride. Some only take out chlorine, lead, etc.

Next, shop for the dried goods you'll be using for the

recipes: sunflower seeds, lentils, mung beans, brown rice, etc. Also nuts (but not peanuts, as these do not feature in the diet) and the Hunza apricots. Bought in fairly large quantities, all these goods can be stored indefinitely and cut down on future shopping expeditions.

With regards to the Hunza apricots, don't be put off by the look of these. They are delicious. And so they should be, grown in the selenium-rich soils of the Himalayas and dried in pure sunshine!

One simple way to get at those all-important apricot kernels is to take the 'stones' from the stewed fruit and put them in a transparent plastic bag. Put this on a hard surface and break open the 'stones' with a tack-hammer. Then open up the bag and take out the kernels to use with the stewed fruit in your breakfast muesli.

Together with sprouted beans, these apricot kernels are the richest source of B-17 in the diet.

As you look through the diets, you'll notice the reference to 'cold-pressed oil'. This is vegetable oil which has been extracted without extra heat or processing. It is therefore particularly pure, and the one for you to use in your diet. But remember to keep it refrigerated, as it goes rancid quite quickly. And a test for rancidity – even when the oil appears to taste all right – is if it goes white in the fridge.

Yoghurt is the only exception to the 'no dairy foods' rule. The best you can buy is made with goat's milk. Added to recipes yoghurt makes them more interesting, but limit helpings to three dessertspoons daily.

Now, if you've also got your vitamin supplements to hand, you're all set to get started on this health-giving programme.

Add a Dash of Ingenuity!

The salad recipes should always be the first course of every meal, freshly prepared and eaten soon afterwards. And salads need never be boring if you try putting them together with a touch of ingenuity.

Add uncooked runner beans, baby broad beans or tender new peapods – all delicious and potassium-rich; or how about tiny florets of raw cauliflower, cubes of apple, a few raisins or fresh grapes? There are so many ways to add interest and unusual textures to salads, remembering that a nutritious vegetable balance consists of including root, stem, leaf and stalk on the plate at the same time. And, of course, don't forget large helpings of beansprouts.

These above all cleanse the bloodstream of impurities and create the alkaline conditions which enhance the action of pancreatic enzymes on the stubborn coating of cancer cells.

In fact, only two vegetables should be avoided since recent studies indicate that parsnips and celery contain substances called psoralens which can cause cancer.

Worse Means Better!

There's an old saying: 'When you put order into chaos, you get more chaos until the new order has time to stabilise.'

Changing to a diet charged with nutrients is a shock to the damaged system. Initially, you'll probably lose weight and, as your body begins to shed the toxins which have suppressed its immune efficiency, find yourself plagued by irritability, flatulence, bad breath, aches and pains, and skin blemishes. Don't worry! These will soon pass. This is just nature's way of indicating that beyond a doubt the diet is working.

SUGGESTED MENUS

Once you know the principles you can experiment to make
varied and appetising meals. To start off with, the following
may prove helpful.

Monday

Breakfast:	Muesli with sesame seeds, buckwheat, wheat-germ, fresh peaches, apple juice
	Slices of wholemeal bread or toast
	Banana and tahini spread
	Peppermint tea (A wide selection of herb teas is available from health food shops, loose or in bags.)
Mid-morning:	Sliced apple
	Fresh fruit juice or herb tea
Lunch:	Fresh carrot juice
	Salad of grated raw beetroot, courgette, lettuce, mung bean sprouts, carrot
	Wholemeal bread
	Orange and banana surprise
Mid-afternoon:	Wholemeal bread with apple and almond spread
	Rose-hip tea
Dinner:	Mixed salad of grated carrot, cauliflower, onion and radish
	Savoury brown rice with chopped nuts
	Wholemeal bread
	Spinach soup
	Fresh fruit salad
Bedtime:	Fresh apple juice

Tuesday

Breakfast:	Cooked buckwheat, millet, barley cereal with fresh orange juice
	Slices of wholemeal bread or toast

	Apple and nut spread
	Camomile tea
Mid-morning:	Banana
	Fresh carrot juice
Lunch:	Salad of mixed beansprouts, grated courgette and lettuce
	Wholemeal bread
	Lentil and onion soup
	Apple and grapefruit cocktail
Mid-afternoon:	Banana and tahini spread on wholemeal bread
	Peppermint tea
Dinner:	Fresh carrot juice
	Salad of alfalfa sprouts, lettuce and fresh herbs
	Baked jacket potato
	Grapes
Bedtime:	Rosemary tea

Wednesday

Breakfast:	Muesli with a little goat's milk yoghurt, fresh pears and grapes
	Slices of wholemeal bread or toast
	Fresh sage and lemon tea
Mid-morning:	Fresh apple juice
Lunch:	Salad of chopped lettuce, cabbage, beansprouts, beetroot or spinach leaves, fresh chives, mint sprinkled with 6 chopped hazel nuts
	Wholemeal bread
	Onion and carrot soup sprinkled with brewer's yeast powder
	Apricot and yoghurt fool
Mid-afternoon:	Rose-hip tea
	Slice of wholemeal bread with banana and orange spread
Dinner:	Large portion of brown rice salad, grated beetroot, sliced onion and chopped walnuts
	Apple and wheatgerm surprise
Bedtime:	Elderflower tea with $\frac{1}{2}$ teaspoon honey and lemon juice to taste

Thursday

Breakfast:	Cooked cereal (millet or oat porridge) with fresh orange and grapefruit segments
	Wholemeal bread or toast with apple, almond and tahini spread
	Mint tea
Mid-morning:	Fresh fruit juice or herb tea
	Apple
Lunch:	Green salad of beansprouts etc.
	Leek and potato soup
	Wholemeal bread
	Fresh fruit
Mid-afternoon:	Camomile tea (with lemon juice if liked)
	Banana
Dinner:	Fresh apple juice
	Large portion of coleslaw
	Cooked brown rice with onion, nuts and herbs
	Baked apple
Bedtime:	Lemon and thyme tea

Friday

Breakfast:	Muesli with a little goat's milk yoghurt, grated apple and fresh orange segments
	Wholemeal bread or toast with tahini spread
	Peppermint tea
Mid-morning:	Fresh carrot and orange juice
	Apple
Lunch:	Salad of beansprouts, chopped cabbage, orange pieces and chopped hazelnuts
	Spiced vegetable soup with sprinkling of brewer's yeast powder
	Wholemeal bread
	Raspberry and yoghurt fool (when in season)
Mid-afternoon:	Rose-hip tea
	Fresh pear
Dinner:	Salad of chopped peppers, onion, lettuce and fresh herbs
	Wholemeal bread

Mixed bean stew

Apple mousse

Bedtime: Lemon balm tea

Saturday

Breakfast: Cooked cereal with fresh sliced pears and grapes

Wholemeal bread or toast with banana and orange spread

Rose-hip tea

Mid-morning: Fresh carrot and apple juice

Lunch: Salad of beansprouts and greenstuff as liked, sprinkled with chopped walnuts

Creamed onion soup

Wholemeal bread

Apricot and yoghurt fool

Rest of the day: Vary your menu according to taste

Sunday

Breakfast: Museli with soaked dried apricots and apple juice

Wholemeal bread or toast with $\frac{1}{2}$ tsp honey

Mint tea

Mid-morning: Fresh apple juice

Lunch: Large portion of green salad using beansprouts etc.

Wholemeal bread

Baked vegetable casserole with tahini and coriander sauce

Watercress (or lettuce) soup

Fresh fruit

Mid-afternoon: Rose-hip tea

Dinner: Fresh carrot, parsley and apple juice mixed

Dandelion salad with humus

Winter borsch soup

Wholemeal bread

Orange and Banana surprise

Bedtime: Peppermint tea

RECIPES

MUESLI

Avoid buying ready-mixed muesli. This is often pre-cooked and may contain sugar and milk powder. Use an organically grown muesli base with as many grains in it as possible. Your healthfood shop will advise you. Add some roughly crushed buckwheat, sesame seeds, sunflower seeds and wheatgerm (this contains oil, so keep it tightly packaged in the fridge), some raisins and/or currants.

Add water until the grain is just covered and leave to soak overnight in a warm place. In the morning (or when the muesli is required) add grated almonds and other nuts, a few pumpkin seeds and a little fruit juice or fresh fruit according to availability. Soya milk and a little honey can be added.

(At some point in your daily diet you should take either kelp powder sprinkled into soup, or kelp tablets which can be bought at the healthfood shops. This adds the trace element iodine to your diet which is necessary for healthy thyroid function.)

COOKED CEREAL (PORRIDGE)

$\frac{1}{2}$ tbs whole buckwheat
$\frac{1}{2}$ tbs Jumbo oats
$\frac{1}{2}$ tbs whole millet
$\frac{1}{2}$ tbs flaked wheat or barley or rye

Soak ingredients overnight (water to cover). Next morning simmer over a low heat until thick. Add extra water if necessary. Eat with fresh fruit and a little yoghurt.

TAHINI AND BANANA SPREAD

Put one ripe banana and 1 tbs tahini (sesame seed paste) into blender. Add lemon juice to taste and 1 tsp sunflower seed oil. Blend until smooth. Use as a spread on wholemeal toast or bread.

For variety try adding a few chopped almonds or a teaspoon of buckwheat to give a crunchy consistency.

APPLE AND ALMOND SPREAD

Put roughly chopped apple into blender with a few almonds and raisins. Blend until smooth. Add a little tahini and 1 tsp safflower oil and lemon juice to taste.

WHOLEMEAL BREAD

You can buy this in your local wholefood or healthfood shop or make your own. A quick method is the 'Grant Loaf' which takes only one hour. The delicious smell in the kitchen will make this well worthwhile!

2 oz (50gm) fresh yeast
2 tsp brown sugar or honey
1¼ pints (750ml) tepid water (more if necessary)
3lbs (1.3kg) 100 per cent stoneground wholewheat flour

Cream yeast with honey or sugar. Add a little warm water and leave until it starts to bubble. Stir into the flour. Add remaining warm water and knead until all the water is taken up. Cover bowl with damp teacloth and leave to rise in a warm place for about 15 minutes.

Divide dough into three and put on slightly oiled baking tins. Put into oven 275-300°F (150°C) gas 2 until bread has risen over top of tins. Then turn oven heat up to 400°F (200°C) gas 6 and bake for about 35 minutes. When the bread is cooked it sounds hollow when you tap it.

Wrap loaves and store in the freezer to use when needed.

FRESH FRUIT AND VEGETABLE JUICES

Pure, undiluted grape juice can be bought from good healthfood shops and kept in the fridge. Otherwise all fruit juices are freshly pressed. Also vegetable juices.

You will gradually be able to judge how much fruit and/or vegetables to put in to get the amount of juice needed. 4 to 6 glasses of carrot juice which is needed daily, takes approximately 7lb (3kg) carrots.

Wash salads and scrub root vegetables but don't peel them more than necessary. The goodness is in the skins. Some people enjoy a mix of grated root vegetables with green leaf and beansprout salads, others prefer to eat them separately.

COLESLAW

$\frac{1}{2}$ lb (225gm) hard cabbage
1 medium apple
1 medium carrot
1 medium onion

Shred finely and mix together with the following dressing:

1 dsp oil
1 sprig chopped borage or parsley
2 tsp lemon juice or cider vinegar
2 comfrey leaves (chopped)

Add a little water or yoghurt and mix.

RED CABBAGE AND ORANGE SALAD

Peel and cut into small pieces $\frac{1}{2}$ an orange. Juice the other half. Finely chop $\frac{1}{2}$lb (225gm) red cabbage. Add fresh chives and parsley, mix with orange pieces and dress with juice.

SPROUTED ALFALFA SALAD

2 tbs sprouted alfalfa seed
1 tsp chopped chives
1 medium grated carrot
½ bunch chopped watercress

Mix with a little lemon juice and oil.

DANDELION SALAD

Chop one good handful of young and tender dandelion leaves (not
gathered from anywhere which might have been sprayed with
chemicals), thoroughly washed
A few chopped spring onions or chives
½ bunch of watercress, rough chopped
1 tbs chopped fresh parsley

Mix with lemon and oil dressing.

SPANISH SALAD

1 onion, thinly sliced
some chopped chicory
a few crisp lettuce leaves
1 orange chopped into pieces
1 tsp chopped fresh mint

Mix with lemon and oil dressing and serve on bed of lettuce.

SWEET POTATO SALAD

Boil 1lb (450gm) sweet potatoes (scrubbed but not peeled). Chop
into cubes. While still warm, dress with the following:

2 tsp oil
1 tbs lemon juice or wine vinegar
1 medium onion, finely chopped
1 clove garlic, crushed

Cool and serve sprinkled with chopped fresh parsley or lemon balm.

WINTER SALAD

Chopped lettuce
1 medium grated carrot
$\frac{1}{2}$ beetroot, grated

Mix with preferred dressing and serve on a bed of chopped watercress.

FENNEL SALAD

1 good-sized bulb of fennel (when in season)
1 large eating apple or 1 peeled orange rough chopped

Wash, slice and mix with lemon juice dressing and serve on a bed of shredded cabbage and/or spinach leaves.

STUFFED PEAR SALAD

$\frac{1}{2}$ ripe dessert pear
little lemon juice
2 tsp sunflower seeds
$\frac{1}{2}$ avocado pear
pinch of ginger

Mash avocado with lemon juice, ginger, sunflower seeds and pear. Pile back into avocado shell and decorate with halved grapes.

CARROT AND ORANGE SALAD

Grate two carrots. Peel and chop 1 orange. Mix together with 2-3 dsps orange juice. Add grated nutmeg or soaked caraway seeds to taste.

BEETROOT AND APPLE SALAD

Finely grate 1 small beetroot and an equal amount of grated apple. Sprinkle with nutmeg, cumin or caraway seeds (previously soaked for one hour in warm water). Add a little grated onion and carrot, fresh horseradish or a pinch of ginger.

(How you flavour these grated salads will eventually be a matter for personal preference.)

FRESH SPINACH SALAD

Wash and chop a handful of spinach leaves. Peel and chop 1 orange. Chop 1 dsp almonds. Mix with a little yoghurt and sprinkle with dill (fresh or dried).

GREEN SALAD

Use any or all of any of the following as available: lettuce, spinach, cabbage, beansprouts, beetroot leaves, watercress, chicory, young turnip tops, etc.

Mix in chopped chives and/or spring onions and parsley. Dress with oil, wine vinegar and crushed garlic *or* plain orange juice *or* small amount of yoghurt with a dash of lemon juice.

ASPARAGUS THE TURKISH WAY

This is costly and seasonal. Keep it for a special treat.

Cut asparagus into bite-size pieces and boil until soft. Drain but keep the liquid to add to juiced drinks. Whilst still warm, arrange asparagus in a dish, pour over Yoghurt Dressing 1 (see over page) and garnish with chopped dill, and/or chives. Tarragon adds a delicious 'bite' to the sauce.

YOGHURT DRESSING 1

Mix the following:

1 tbs yoghurt
1 onion, finely chopped
1 clove garlic, crushed
1 tsp lemon juice

YOGHURT DRESSING 2

Mix or liquidise the following:

1 tbs yoghurt
1 clove garlic, crushed
$\frac{1}{2}$ tsp fresh tarragon (if dried, soak in lemon juice for 1 hour)
$\frac{1}{4}$ tsp paprika (or more to taste)

LEMON AND OIL DRESSING

Mix 1 tbs lemon juice and 2 tbs safflower or sunflower seed oil (cold-pressed).

SPINACH SOUP

Make a paste with 2 teaspoons cold-pressed oil and 1 dessertspoon wholemeal flour. Warm in a pan and add enough water and/or vegetable stock to make a thin, creamy consistency. Chop two handfuls of spinach leaves and cook in the sauce for three to five minutes or until just tender. Remove from heat and put through blender.

This soup can also be made with any other green leaf vegetable and cauliflower if chopped into small pieces before cooking.

Sprinkle with finely chopped onion or parsley.

LENTIL AND ONION SOUP

3oz (75gm) lentils
1 tsp oil
1 carrot, chopped
¾ pt (450ml) water or stock
1 medium onion, sliced into rings
1 bay leaf, crushed garlic, chopped chives or parsley, according to taste.

Wash lentils. Cook in water and oil for about 10 minutes. Add chopped vegetables. Bring to the boil and simmer gently until tender. Add more water if necessary. Serve with a little lemon juice stirred into soup and sprinkled with chopped parsley or chives etc.
   (If preferred, this soup can be blended smooth.)

ONION AND CARROT SOUP

1 large onion
2 medium carrots
left-over cooked brown rice, if available

Chop vegetables and cook in water until tender. Add a little milk (if allowed) and serve sprinkled with brewer's yeast powder and chopped parsley.

LEEK AND POTATO SOUP

1 large leek
1 medium potato with skin
Sunflower seeds

Chop vegetables. Boil until tender. Add sunflower seeds and liquidise in blender. Serve sprinkled with brewer's yeast and chopped chives.

BAKED SWEET POTATOES

These are not related to ordinary potatoes but are cooked in the same way. Wash and bake in their skins and serve with a vegetable casserole or a salad mixed with yoghurt dressing.

LEEK AND JERUSALEM ARTICHOKE SOUP

Stir-fry in a little good oil: 1 leek, 2 or 3 artichokes and 2 carrots, all chopped. Add one pint (600ml) vegetable stock, 1 bay leaf, 1 clove garlic, crushed and a little basil. Simmer until tender. Liquidise and serve sprinkled with dill.

SPICED VEGETABLE SOUP

1 medium onion
2 medium carrots
1 leek
1 turnip or swede (small ones)
a little cabbage

Chop the vegetables and cook in water until just tender. Add a teaspoon each of aniseed, marjoram and dill. Liquidise and serve sprinkled with brewer's yeast powder and chopped parsley.

BAKED VEGETABLE CASSEROLE WITH TAHINI AND CORIANDER SAUCE

Chop: 1 medium onion, 1 leek, 1 carrot, 2 Jerusalem artichokes. Place in a casserole with a little water and bake at 350°F (180°C) gas 4 until tender. Make a sauce with wholemeal flour and oil and liquid from casserole. Add a little lemon juice, 1 level tbs tahini and pour over casserole. Serve hot.

VEGETABLE CASSEROLE

Chop: 1 medium carrot, stick of celery, 1 onion, $\frac{1}{2}$ cooking apple. Add 2 dessertspoons brown lentils, 1 tsp each of sage and thyme and 1 dessertspoon oats for thickening. Cover with water or vegetable stock and bake at 350°F (180°C) gas 4, in a tight-fitting casserole until tender.

ROAST VEGETABLE CASSEROLE

Scrub and chop the following: 1 sweet potato, 1 leek, 1 carrot, 1 artichoke, 1 onion. Par-boil (about 10 minutes) and place in an oiled oven dish. Chop three cloves of garlic and quickly sauté in a little oil. Pour over vegetables and roast in the oven until tender. Serve with lentil sauce.

LENTIL SAUCE

Cook a quantity of green lentils with some carrots, onions, turnip and garlic. When soft, purée in liquidiser, adding dill, basil and sage or fresh mint. (If necessary, thicken with wholemeal flour.)

CREAMED ONION SOUP

Boil 8oz (225gm) chopped onion until tender. Heat a little oil in a saucepan and add 1 tbs wholemeal flour. Stir in onion and add more water to give a creamy consistency. Liquidise and serve hot, sprinkled with brewer's yeast and chopped fresh parsley.

STUFFED MARROW

Halve a marrow, scoop out seeds and fill with: 1 peeled and chopped onion, a few chopped mushrooms, 1 clove garlic, crushed, 2-3 tbs brown breadcrumbs or 2 tbs millet seed cooked until tender. Add 1 tbs of ground almonds and a little thyme.

Wrap in foil and bake in an oven-proof dish with a little water, until tender.

WINTER BORSCH

1 dsp oil, in which sauté the following: 1 large grated beetroot, 1 chopped onion, 1 chopped carrot, a small red cabbage (about 1lb/450gm), chopped.

Cover with water and simmer until vegetables are just tender. Add ½ cup of puréed tomatoes, chopped fresh (or dried) dill and parsley. Stir in a sprinkling of brewer's yeast powder and a spoonful of yoghurt just before serving.

Brown rice is always used in rice recipes. It has a better flavour than white rice and because it is unpolished, the covering of the seeds is rich in B Vitamins, Iron and Calcium. Brown rice takes a little longer to cook, has a nutty flavour and should not be rinsed before serving.

SAVOURY BROWN RICE

1 cup of brown rice
1 large onion
1 tsp mixed herbs or sage (fresh if possible)
1 cup boiling water
1 tsp oil
2oz (50gm) mushrooms
1 tbs cucumber, chopped

Wash rice. Chop vegetables. Bring water to the boil and add other ingredients. Simmer gently with the lid on the pan for 30 minutes. For variety, add sunflower seeds, raisins and dill seeds.

RICE SALAD

Boil one cup of rice in 1 cup of water with 1 bay leaf and a little rosemary. When cooked, cool and dress with a little oil, cider vinegar, chopped fresh parsley and chives or raw chopped onion. Apricots which have been soaked overnight can be chopped and added for additional flavour.

RICE WITH HERBS

Instead of cooking the rice as above, boil with bay leaf and add freshly chopped rosemary, sage, chives, lemon balm and parsley when it has cooled. Dress if liked with a little cider vinegar, oil and garlic dressing.

RICE PILAFF

1 cup of rice
1 sliced bell pepper (red or green)
1 sliced leek
1 medium onion, chopped
2oz (50gm) chopped sultanas or apricots

Boil in water (1 to $1\frac{1}{2}$ cups) until tender. Serve with a dressing of 1 tsp oil and chopped hazelnuts or almonds.

Pulse, nuts, seeds and yoghurt all contain protein to provide the anti-cancer diet with correctly balanced nourishment.

HUMUS

$\frac{1}{2}$lb (225gm) chickpeas, soaked overnight. Cook in same water until tender and then liquidise.
   Add the following: 2 cloves of garlic, crushed, 2-3 tbs tahini, 4 tbs oil. Liquidise again and serve with salads or as a sandwich spread. Humus will keep in a covered container in the fridge.

MIXED BEAN STEW

1 dsp each butter beans, haricot beans, wholewheat and mung

beans. Soak ingredients overnight (soak mung beans separately). Discard water and rinse. Mung beans take about 20 minutes to cook; the remainder take about 35 minutes. Either cook mung beans separately or add to the others 15 minutes after they have been cooking. Add a chopped onion, crushed garlic and a bay leaf to add flavour. Serve hot with a sprinkling of oil and brewer's yeast or serve cold with a salad.

NUT ROAST

2oz (50gm) cashew nuts
1 large onion
4oz (100gm) fresh brown breadcrumbs (or cooked millet)
3 level tbs soya flour mixed with sage or rosemary to flavour
2oz (50gm) walnuts
1 large carrot
a little oil

Sauté finely chopped onion and carrot. Mill the nuts. Add crumbs (or millet), herbs, garlic, etc. and mix. Place in an oiled glass or earthenware casserole or a baking tin lined with tinfoil. Sprinkle with sesame seeds and a little oil. Bake at 350°F (180°C) gas 4 for 30-40 minutes or until browned.

FRUIT AND YOGHURT FOOL

Use any fresh fruits as available. Grate or mash, add 2 tbs yoghurt and liquidise. Serve sprinkled with chopped almonds, walnuts or sesame seeds.

Suggested fruits: soaked or fresh apricots, prunes, raspberries, blackberries, peaches, apples, bananas, oranges, pears, plums, grapes. Approximately 4oz (100gm) fruit to 2 tbs yoghurt.

ORANGE AND BANANA SURPRISE

Liquidise 1 peeled orange, 1 banana with a little lemon juice and serve chilled and sprinkled with a few sultanas and sesame seeds.

APPLE AND GRAPEFRUIT

Roughly chop one unpeeled dessert apple with the segments of half
a grapefruit. Mix and serve with a few grapes.

APPLE AND WHEATGERM

Grate one medium dessert apple (with skin) and add a little
orange or lemon juice. Sprinkle on ½ tsp chopped, fresh rosemary.
Mix in 1 tsp wheatgerm and 1 tsp toasted sunflower seeds.
  (Sunflower seeds can be toasted by placing a small quantity in
a dry iron or stainless steel saucepan and shaking over a medium
heat until they begin to brown.)

BAKED APPLE

Take a large cooking apple and remove the core. Grind the pips
with ½ tbs walnuts, ½ tbs cinnamon, ½ tbs coriander and 1 tbs
sultanas or currants. Pour over apple and bake until just soft.

APPLE MOUSSE

Liquidise two sweet apples (with skins), add a little lemon juice,
ginger and nutmeg or cinnamon. Serve sprinkled with sesame
seeds (toasted if liked) and chopped almonds.

HOME-MADE YOGHURT

If yoghurt is new to you, don't expect to like it immediately. It is
an acquired taste.
  The trick of making yoghurt is to keep it warm until it thickens.
You can buy an electric yoghurt maker to do this, or you can use
a wide-necked thermos. As it is probable that cow's milk will have
traces of penicillin which may prevent the yoghurt from
thickening, if you can get goat's milk this is the best milk to use.
  You will need a kitchen thermometer and a little commercial

yoghurt to 'start' the milk. Or you can buy Yoghurt Culture from healthfood shops with the instructions on the packet.

Heat 1 pint (600ml) milk to boiling and then allow to cool to 37°C. Place two tsp of commercial yoghurt into the thermos, pour in cooled milk and mix thoroughly. Cork the thermos and leave until the yoghurt has thickened. This takes from five to seven hours. Then keep in the fridge and use as required.

The next batch of yoghurt is made by using two teaspoonfuls of the previous one but don't make more than three or four batches of yoghurt in this way. The yoghurt bacteria becomes weakened and a new 'strain' is needed after every three or four successive batches of yoghurt. Remember to take very little yoghurt. Milk has growth factors in it.

Catering for the Cancer Patient within the Family

It is to be hoped that the patient following the anti-cancer diet can depend upon the support and encouragement of the rest of the family. Keeping to a strict diet when the rest of the family is eating different foods may mean preparing two lots of food at every meal, but when the family understands the importance of what the patient is doing to help him or herself get well again, then they can add loving-care-and-kindness to the anti-cancer menu. Then, perseverance is the name of the game.

Some Important Do's and Don'ts

Do eat frequent small meals rather than have large and infrequent ones.
Do eat slowly and chew your food well to aid digestion.
Do take time to eat in pleasant surroundings.
Do throw away left-over foods. Fresh is best.
Don't drink with meals. This dilutes and washes valuable

GIVE UP	REASON WHY	CHANGE TO
Alcohol except no more than 2 glasses of wine per day	Your liver is already overworked and exhausted in the effort to eliminate disease	*Any* fresh fruit or vegetable juice
Smoking	Is a proven carcinogenic destroys vital Vitamin C	No substitute
Coffee, Tea, Chocolate	Are stimulants which also burden the liver	Herb teas. Highland Spring water, Slippery Elm
Meat, Poultry, Fish, Shellfish	The enzymes required to digest these proteins are the ones your body needs to break down cancer cells	Beans, nuts and sprouting grains (Not peanuts)
Salt	Destroys the potassium/sodium balance essential for good health, affects the adrenals and creates stress	Kelp, Ruthmol (salty-tasting substitute – obtainable from healthfood shops), fresh garlic, herbs
Sugar	Uses up precious B vitamins and calcium, and disturbs gastro-intestinal tract	Strictly limited amounts of honey, maple syrup, blackstrap molasses. For special treats only
Butter, Cheese, Eggs, Milk, Cream, Margarine	Too much fat content	Soy milk, very small amounts of cheese and butter occasionally for a treat
All canned, smoked, bottled, preserved, manufactured, and synthetic products and flavourings	Dead food has no value and the additives are positively harmful	Fresh, raw, home made foods and beverages

nutrients through the system before they can be properly absorbed.

Don't skip meals. Every mouthful counts.

Do crack open the stones of fresh apricots, peaches, plums, cherries etc. and eat the kernels with the fruit. These seeds are rich in B-17. Similarly, when eating apples, eat the pips as well. These also are rich in nitrilosides. *Don't* add extra bran to your diet. Bran is a hard fibre and too much upsets the bowels. There is plenty of bran and soft fibre in the diet. Additions are quite unnecessary.

The table on page 125 is an easy way to remember the items which must be avoided. But there is one small change to the embargo on alcohol. If the patient chooses, two small glasses of dry, white wine a day or two small tots of spirits can be taken. This is thought to stimulate the disease-fighting substances called prostaglandins.

Let the Light Shine In

The eye as the window of the soul may be poetic fancy, but it is a fact that the eyes are the windows to two important glands in the body, both programmed by nature to function in response to the *full spectrum* daylight entering the eyes. These are the pineal and pituitary glands, which control healthy hormone function.

Artificial lighting – or light which comes through glass – is not the same as natural daylight. It lacks the benefit of ultraviolet rays; certainly too much exposure to this light can be harmful, but equally certain, too little will deprive the body of proper stimulation.

So get out in the natural light whenever you can, without wearing ordinary glasses or sunglasses.

Pure sunlight – like pure water – is essential for health.

8 METABOLIC THERAPY FOR TUMOUR DESTRUCTION

'It's very important to realise that this therapy does not work unless you have already decided to follow the diet,' says Dr Alec Forbes, medical director. 'It's true that the Diet alone can control some cancers, but the addition of Metabolic Therapy greatly improves the results. The Psychological and Healing aspects are equally important. We are talking about a total therapy. The separate regimes are combined to make up the whole approach.

'Orthodox cancer specialists have not used or researched this therapy. Therefore they can truthfully make remarks such as: "There is no evidence that patients benefit from this approach, except emotionally"; or "There is no evidence that it works." Their knowledge is mostly limited to scientific journals. If time does not permit them to read more widely, they may understandably adopt a sceptical attitude towards this new approach for cancer control. The only acceptable yardstick is whether or not it works. We have plenty of evidence to show that this is what counts for many of the people who choose to follow the gentle way.

'Dr Hans Nieper has researched the non-toxic metabolic therapy in great depth. English translations of his papers on cancer treatment can be obtained from the A. Keith Brewer Library, Richland Centre, Wisconsin 53581, USA. It is a rapidly advancing field and links with it are now appearing in orthodox medical research concerned with reversing genetic cancer by metabolic means. [D.F. Horrobin, *Medical Hypotheses*, 1980.]

'Moreover, numerous doctors throughout the world have been independently following non-toxic therapy methods and have observed that patients who have failed to respond to orthodox cancer treatments have made a good recovery when using Metabolic Therapy methods.

'The substances used in this therapy are mostly obtainable from the Healthfood industry where there is a wide range of quality and purity depending upon the source of supply. In general terms, a high price does not necessarily guarantee the best quality. On the other hand, where Amygdalin is concerned, the best quality does cost more.'

The substances used in non-toxic metabolic cancer therapy are harmless in the doses given here.

The co-operation of a sympathetic NHS medical practitioner may enable the patient to get all the items mentioned on prescription.

The Programme

1. Metabolic Therapy is designed to take the patient through several stages of detoxification. This means that from between four to seven days after beginning the programme, the cancer tumours will begin to break down and be carried into the bloodstream for elimination in the normal way. At this time the patient will have a reaction (toxaemia). This indicates that the therapy is succeeding although the patient will perhaps feel unwell.

When toxic symptoms occur, some of the given substances are reduced or withdrawn until the reaction subsides. Liver stimulation is increased by enemas, especially if there is vomiting. Then they are resumed. If toxic symptoms persist, reduced dosage may be necessary.

For instance, if after five days the patient displays symptoms of toxicity, the amount of Amygdalin given at the onset of these symptoms should be noted and then withheld until symptoms subside. Then the patient starts taking Amygdalin again beginning with the dose at a slightly lower level than the one which was given at the onset of the reaction. This is called the threshold dose and only applies to Amygdalin, Vitamin A and the Pancreatic Enzyme

Tablets. The other substances in the programme are continued at regular daily doses.

2. Toxaemia (feverishness, headaches, the 'shivers', a sense of depression) is an indication that the liver is not coping with the extra load imposed by the elimination of the toxic products of damaged cancer cells. But it is not desirable to get rid of the tumours more quickly than the liver can work. That is why with Amygdalin, Vitamin A and Pancreatic Enzymes, a short rest period is sometimes given after each bout of toxaemia, before resuming treatment at the previous threshold dosages. This short period should be no more than a day or two.

3. Enemas of liver herbs or coffee should be taken when there is excessive breakdown of cancer tumours as these help the liver to flush toxins from the body. (Instructions on pages 137-8.)

4. The effectiveness of Metabolic Therapy relies on the adjustment of the given substances. Insufficient doses will fail to produce toxaemia; too much will burden the patient's system with more destroyed cancer cells than the liver can comfortably deal with. This emphasises the need for a disciplined and, when possible, skilled approach to this therapy method. Every person is unique and has different requirements.

5. When the Metabolic Therapy programme does not produce further symptoms of detoxification, the patient will experience a renewed sense of wellbeing. It can then be assumed that the tumours have been successfully dissolved and one or other of the diagnostic tests which originally established the presence of cancer, may confirm this.

6. BCG (Tuberculosis vaccine) is often given after one month on the Metabolic Therapy and thereafter at intervals of five weeks to twelve weeks until the patient has responded

to the therapy. (This is to act as a stimulating agent to the patient's sluggish natural defence system.)

7.   Daily injections (and/or oral doses) of Amygdalin form an important part of this therapy, but *only if the patient is committed to the diet*. Amygdalin works best in conjunction with the diet and other vitamin and mineral substances, which are *bonded together into a strict daily routine*. NB GPs can prescribe Amygdalin. If in doubt, contact The Family Practitioners' Advisory Committee or the DHSS.

8.   When ordering the substances listed on the following pages, the patient should obtain at least 14 days' supplies in advance to ensure that the daily doses are continued without a break. Once contact has been established with a reputable supplier, orders can usually be made by telephone but as some substances come from abroad, the patient should make sure of having sufficient doses to compensate for delayed arrival.

Substances with a Direct Action on Cancer Cells

VITAMIN A

The best source is freshly prepared carrot juice emulsified by whisking with a teaspoonful of vegetable oil (preferably cold-pressed) in a liquidiser and drunk as soon as possible. This contains B-carotene which is more effective and less toxic than commercial Vitamin A. Work the dose up rapidly to four to six 4oz (150ml) glasses a day (about $1\frac{1}{2}$ pints (900ml) per day.) Monitor the dose level. There should be marked yellow staining of the hands without a headache. Whenever a steady headache occurs – reduce the daily intake by half as tolerance improves.

  All Vitamin A that is not emulsified, goes directly to the liver where it is stored. Emulsifying Vitamin A enables it to circulate in adequate amounts at the site of the cancer cells where it releases the protein digesting enzyme which de-shields them. Emulsified Vitamin A and Carotene are absorbed in the lymphatic system and so bypass the liver.

B-Carotene is also available in capsules and can, on the advice of the therapist, be substituted for fresh carrot juice.

AMYGDALIN

Patients who elect not to have the *full programme* of metabolic substances should *not* take Amygdalin (also referred to as Laetrile/B-17/nitrilosides). This substance is expensive and does not give good results when used on its own. To be effective, Amygdalin requires large quantities of Vitamin A and the correct administration of enzyme retention enemas and supplements at strategic intervals. Then Amygdalin plays an important part in tumour destruction.

Amygdalin can be taken either by injection or in tablet form. The former route is usually more effective, especially in controlling metastases and subduing pain. However, it must be said that results obtained with Amygdalin will depend upon the type of cancer, the quality of supplies, and the patient's own ability to observe the co-ordinated wholistic approach as explained throughout this book. Then the dosage is as follows:

Start with one 2.5gm ampoule and work up to 2 or 3 ampoules daily, given in one injection half an hour *after* the patient has taken a Wobe Mugos Retention enema.

After three weeks reduce to bi-weekly injections and on other days of the week take oral doses of D-Amygdalin tablets. Oral dose is 240mg three times daily on an empty stomach and with *not less* than a four-hour interval between doses, or between the injections and oral doses. If using 500 mg tablets, take one tablet one day and two tablets the next.

ENZYMES

Enzymes should be taken before Amygdalin. They de-shield the cancer cells and prepare them for destruction by the chemical break down of Amygdalin at the site of the tumour. (See Chapter 5.)

Amygdalin frequently eases the pain from secondary cancers. Sometimes the patient will ache a little after taking Amygdalin, but this is a good sign and soon passes.

BENZALDEHYDE

These capsules containing 100 mgm of Benzaldehyde in oil can be taken three times daily as well as Amygdalin and are also available on prescription. In addition to blocking the fermentation action of cancer cells, it also helps with any pain. Benzaldehyde is also useful in cases of brain tumours as it penetrates the blood-brain barrier which Amygdalin does not. Take Benzaldehyde on an empty stomach with doses of Amygdalin. Benzaldehyde should be taken with not less than half a glass of water, preferably spring water.

MAGNESIUM

Dolomite tablets contain 300mg Calcium Carbonate and 200mg Magnesium Carbonate. Take 5 tablets daily as treatment and 3 tablets daily for maintenance later on.

These are cheaper than the orotates.

MAGNESIUM OROTATE

Take 500mg twice daily.

CALCIUM OROTATE

Take 500mg twice daily. Always take magnesium and calcium together. They balance each other. If you take too much of one, it depresses the level of the other in the body.

POTASSIUM OROTATE

Take 200mg daily. If suffering from diarrhoea, take 600mg daily and reduce when symptom clears.

SELENIUM

Take 200 micrograms twice daily for two months, then reduce to 100 micrograms every other day. Remember only take your Selenium in the form of a compressed tablet of Selenium Yeast which selectively takes up Selenium from the environment and binds it in a form that is easily absorbed.

VITAMIN C

500mg of Calcium Ascorbate with Bioflavinoids in a tablet that is released into the upper part of the small intestine are recommended for better absorption and utilisation. Take 12 500mg tablets spread out over the day and with food. This dose can be increased if the tablets are well tolerated. If ascorbic acid or a very soluble source of Vitamin C is used, there can be diarrhoea or excess acidity in the body which may need a reduction in the dose.

VITAMIN B-COMPLEX

This also helps Amygdalin to work and may be taken as

Brewer's Yeast tablets: 3 tablets three times daily. Also yeast powder (Yestamin) added to soups and muesli. Vitamin B-1 (Thiamine) has a similar effect. Take 3mg three times daily with meals. No other members of the Vitamin B group should be taken. Vitamins B6 and B12 tend to be growth enhancers if taken in excess.

UVA URSI TEA (Mountain Box)

This contains Arbutine which enhances the action of Amygdalin and helps to prevent the formation of scar tissue when tumours have been dissolved.

Infuse 1oz (25gm) leaves to 1 pint (600ml) boiling water. Cool and drink 1 wineglass three times daily.

NB Uva Ursi tea should not be taken continuously. Take it for about two months then drop it from the daily programme for the next month or so. Uva Ursi tea should not be taken at all when kidney disease is present.

Substances that Expose the Cancer Cell for Destruction

ENZYME RETENTION ENEMAS (Wobe Mugos)

Enzyme enemas are taken one to three times daily. Enzymes given by enema bypass the digestive system and are rapidly absorbed into the bloodstream in their most efficient form. As previously explained, protein-digesting enzymes break down the shielding on the cancer cell and expose it for the destructive action of Amygdalin.

The instructions for taking wobe mugos retention enemas are on page 140.

BROMELAIN

This is a concentrate of protein-digesting enzymes extracted from pineapples. Again, the proteolytic enzymes are those which damage the muco-protein covering on cancer cells without harming healthy cells.

Take 100mg tablets four times daily before meals. Increase this dose to 800mg daily gradually over 2 weeks but stop if there are any signs of bleeding. Resume when the bleeding has stopped.

PANCREX V CAPSULES

Take 3 capsules before meals four times daily. Both Bromelain and Pancrex V are taken on an empty stomach in order to get the maximum absorption into the bloodstream. If they are taken with food they will be used to digest food and diverted from the more important work of de-shielding the cancer cells.

Increasing Immunity

The following substances help to build up the damaged immune system in conjunction with The Diet and Supplements as described in Chapters 7 and 8.

VITAMIN D2

Calcium with Vitamin D tablets BPC: take 1 daily. *Crush* before swallowing with meals.

GINSENG

This raises immunity and is a source of natural steroids. Take a 250mg tablet daily.

ZINC OROTATE

15mg daily for maintenance. More if there is a known deficiency. Take with meals.

EVENING PRIMROSE CAPSULES

Take 500mg three times daily. These supply Gamma Linoleic Acid which stimulates the presence of Prostaglandin E1 in the bloodstream. Prostaglandins inhibit the fermenting growth of cancer cells.

FEVER THE HEALER

Most orthodox doctors try to combat and suppress fever. Actually fever is a constructive, health-promoting symptom, initiated and created by the body in its fight to eradicate infections and other conditions of disease. Fever (or high body temperature) speeds the healing process.

At Bristol, after one month on the diet and Vitamin and Mineral Supplements, a further boost to the immune system is given by a doctor with BCG vaccinations. It is best to start with a Heaf Test. If this gives a marked reaction, i.e. Stage 3 or 4, continue with this once a fortnight and when the reaction gets down to Stage 1 or 2, give 0.1ml intradermally at 5 to 12 week intervals. One should wait until the acute inflammatory reaction is dying away and the scar shows signs of healing before giving another dose.

Another way of giving the BCG is 0.1ml diluted in 5ml of sterile saline subcutaneously. This gives a more diffuse instead of a sharp local reaction and can be repeated when the mild inflammatory reaction has practically subsided. This requires more frequent injections than the first method. These injections are continued for some months until the patient's disease has stabilised.

Detoxification

When the treatment is taking effect, many cancer cells are being dissolved into the bloodstream for detoxification by the liver. Unless the liver is functioning efficiently, toxic substances may build up and produce a feeling of collapse. Symptoms of this include fever, fast pulse, sweating and headaches. The liver needs to be stimulated to cleanse the toxins out of the body. This is done with herbs which increase the flow of bile. Coffee enemas may also be helpful if there is vomiting and/or pain.

Patients taking the Metabolic Therapy programme will find that for a month or so at least it will be necessary to suspend all other activities and concentrate on keeping a strict timetable of medicaments, meals, and the meditation exercises explained in Chapter 9.

HERBS FOR LIVER STIMULATION

Barks and Roots

Barbery Bark	15gm
Fringe Tea Bark	40gm
Dandelion Root	75gm
Gentian Root	45gm
Burdock Root	55gm
Echinacea Root	40gm

Leaves

Centaury Herb	60gm
Holy Thistle	30gm

Put 2oz (50gm) of barks and roots into $1\frac{1}{2}$ pints (900ml) of water. Bring to the boil and simmer for 20 minutes. Put 1oz (25gm) leaves into a thermos. Strain the boiling extract of the barks and roots onto the leaves. Leave overnight, strain and refrigerate.

Take 1oz (25gm) of the extract, twice a day. Dilute if desired. Liquid extracts of the herbs in the proportions above can be used instead.

If these herbs are used for liver stimulation, routine coffee enemas can be avoided. The herbs can also be given by an enema in an emergency. Coffee enemas are much used in the USA for liver stimulation and are very effective for this.

Coffee Enemas

Enemas are not something we go in for in this country although abroad they are used much more freely and people take them for granted. So the first thing is to get over the feeling that you are going to do something strange. Enemas are a quick and easy way to clear the system of the poisons which are making you ill. They also help to relieve any pain.

To give yourself enemas you need a gravity feed enema kit which you can probably buy at your local chemist. If not they will be able to give you the name of a supplier.

You will also need ground coffee (fresh or tinned but instant won't do), a piece of plastic sheeting or an old towel, a good supply of mansize tissues, a tube of K-Y Jelly and, for extra comfort, a pillow for your head since you are going to be lying on the floor. Make yourself as comfortable as possible: being thoroughly relaxed is the secret of a successful enema.

HOW TO MAKE THE COFFEE ENEMAS

Add 3 tablespoons of freshly ground coffee to one quart (1.2 litres) water. Boil fast for three minutes then simmer for 15 minutes. Cool and strain.

If you want to make enough for several enemas at the same time, double the coffee content and then dilute with cold water. Always warm to body temperature for the enema. One pint of coffee is needed for each enema.

The bathroom is probably the best place to give yourself an enema. Make sure the rest of the family know you are going to be in there for about 20 minutes so that you will be left undisturbed. Then carefully prepare everything you need.

Cover the floor with the plastic sheet or the old towelling. Arrange your pillow and have a radio or a book to pass the time. A battery timer is useful. If the bathroom is cold, have a rug handy. Fit up the enema kit and hang the container at least two feet above where you are lying. Now you are ready to begin.

1   Pour 1 pint (600ml) of bloodheat coffee into enema container, having first remembered to secure the tap on the tube.
2   Set empty jug on the floor, release the tap on the catheter and allow a little coffee to flow into the jug to make sure all the air is out of the tube.
3   Turn off tap. Empty coffee in the jug back into the enema container.
4   Return jug to floor and put end of catheter into it.
5   Lie on your left side with your knees up, making yourself comfortable.
6   Grease the nozzle of the catheter with a little K-Y jelly.
7   Make a conscious effort to relax your body.
8   When you feel ready, gently push the catheter into the rectum, bearing down as you do so to open the ring of muscle.
9   When the catheter is properly in place, turn on the tap

until you feel the coffee flowing in. Don't let it flow too
fast. Give yourself plenty of time. Hold up the tube to
ease in the last of the coffee.

10   Turn off the tap and remove the catheter which is
replaced in the jug.

11   Massage your stomach to spread the enema.

12   Now relax – listen to the radio or read for the next
fifteen minutes.

Obviously it is easier to take the coffee enemas if you've
emptied your bowels first. A warm water enema to flush out
the colon before taking the coffee enemas, may be a good
idea.

Hold the coffee enema for as long as you can. If 1 pint
(600ml) is, to begin with, too much – work up to this
amount. Once you get used to the procedure, you will find it
remarkably simple.

Although taking coffee enemas is a time-consuming
procedure, you will soon look forward to these sessions
because they make you feel so much better. The coffee is
quickly absorbed into the bloodstream via the veins in the
rectum and then through the portal vein to the liver. There
it stimulates the production of bile which carries waste
substances out of the body in the normal way.

Take coffee enemas whenever you feel the need. If you
are sticking to the Diet and the Metabolic Therapy, your
system is being cleansed of all that has been making you ill.
Coffee enemas speed up this refreshment.

Wobe Mugos Retention Enemas

A retention enema is intended to be held until it is absorbed
so make sure your bowels are empty before taking one. *The
amount of fluid is very small and should present no problems.*

Instructions for making up the retention enemas come

with the kits which are ready to use.

Try to arrange so that the enzyme retention enema is taken in bed last thing at night.

Protein Deficiency

A high protein intake is not necessary except in cases of advanced cancer. Then it is protein deficiency which kills the patient, not the disease. The demands of the cancer tumour for protein lead to the wasting of muscles and organs in the patient's body. The efficiency of the intestine in absorbing food is impaired by lack of protein and so a vicious circle is established.

In such cases high protein supplements are an advantage. PEP (Pure Essential Protein) contains all eight essential amino-acids and more. It is low in salt and of vegetable origin. Thirty to 60 grammes per day sprinkled on food or in drinks is all that is required for a high protein supplement.

Relaxation & Peace of Mind

There are many factors that interfere with the successful application of nutritional and biological therapies, such as toxic environment; ineffective digestion and assimilative system; emotional stresses; anxiety, worries, fears, etc. If the patient is under severe stress or acute anxiety, ability to absorb and utilise nutritional and medical factors will be seriously impaired and the expected healing may not take place until the emotional disturbance is alleviated. The patient must be able to acquire a state of total relaxation and peace of mind to take full advantage of the programme so far described.

Also, the patient should have a thorough understanding of the basic philosophy of biological medicine and of the purpose behind the various diet and supplement routines, so that there is complete confidence in the prescribed methods of treatment and in the part he is asked to play in their administration.

It is Your Body, Your Life

The Metabolic Therapy course only lasts in its first intensive form for one or two months. Some people choose to use it before accepting conventional treatment. There is every argument in favour of trying it before going for conventional treatment other than that needed in an emergency. This time lapse will not be a significant delay if the patient then decides to proceed with conventional treatments. Then the two approaches can be combined.

Orthodox treatment for cancer is always directed at the cancer tumour (the symptoms), not at the whole person who, over a long period, has become ill.

Moreover, orthodox treatments require patients to submit passively to whatever is prescribed. As the reader will by now have realised, biological medicine is largely a self-help programme. The person who wants to regain his or her health is very much involved at every level of treatment, and this is as it should be.

An effective cure for any disease can only be accomplished *from within*. Consequently the first principle of biological medicine is to create conditions most conducive to self-healing; to support, stimulate and activate the body's own healing activity with harmless and effective measures.

The Bristol Diet and the Metabolic Therapy Programme are combined to attack the physical symptoms of cancer. Learning to regenerate other vital self-healing but non-physical energies is explained on the following pages.

Many naturopath therapists consider that these mind-over-matter exercises may well be the key which will open the door to recovery.

9   GATEWAY TO THE GENTLE PATH

The Chinese write the word 'Crisis' with two ideograms; one means 'danger', the other 'opportunity'.

Of course, a confrontation with cancer is a dangerous life crisis. It can also be a much needed opportunity to stop, look and listen quietly to what disease is trying to tell you about yourself and your way of living.

The physical approach to cancer control – by the Diet and vitamin therapy methods, is of extreme importance. However, it is the non-physical aspect of the wholistic therapies which present the patient with the key to the kingdom of change.

As you will have probably realised, following the anti-cancer programme devised at Bristol involves hard work and personal effort. So now you can relax and enjoy what comes next. It is by learning deep relaxation that patients manage to generate the subtle healing pathways of the mind. Once the cancer patient has learnt to relax it is possible to allow healing to happen.

Crisis plus Opportunity means Change

The therapists at the Bristol Cancer Help Centre would be the first to admit that it isn't always easy for patients to recognise cancer as a transformational experience, or to appreciate that although diet is important, vitamin therapy is also important, ultimately it will be the patient's ability to harness natural, self-healing processes which will lay the foundations for the possibility of a new equation: crisis plus opportunity plus change means recovery.

Counselling for Change

The patient's mental outlook is of extreme importance. Self-defeating attitudes need correction by a trained psychotherapist.

Initially, at the first interview at Bristol, Dr Alec uses a system of personality testing which is based on the emotional significance of colour. Called the Luscher Personality Test, patients are asked to select from a chart colours in order of preference. The relative values of each choice and combinations of colours permit a comprehensive assessment of the patient's basic character. Then it is a matter for discussion and gentle probing to enable the patient to come to terms with the deep-seated emotional problems which so often lie at the root of serious ill-health.

It has often been said that disease is the result of an obstruction to the natural energy flow within the body. Remove the obstruction and you remove the disease.

If it were just a matter of using a spiritual Dynarod this would present no problems! Fortunately, at Bristol the therapists have less forceful ways to unblock the obstruction. It is achieved by tender-loving-care-and-kindness and counselling provided by those best qualified to give it because they themselves have a first-hand knowledge of the problems involved.

The sick person is persuaded to come up with some honest answers to some difficult and deeply revealing questions:

'Why has this disease developed in me at this time?'

'What is cancer telling me about my way of life and the kind of person I am?'

'If what I've been doing up to now has led to disease, how can I change?'

Many patients find the answers painful. Honesty often is. But, like forking out the money for an expensive air trip, once the ticket is paid for the passenger can then sit back and enjoy the ride.

Examining deep emotions helps patients identify certain

ingrained behaviour patterns in a lifestyle which may have a lot wrong with it.

The person who is 'using' cancer to gain love and attention formerly lacking in his or her life, needs to be aware of this. Feelings of fear, hopelessness and helplessness are brought out into the open. Frustration, resentment, hostility all have to be understood for what they are: negative emotions which have damned the free-flow of vitality and growth and become a barrier to recovery. Life is growth. Anything less is stagnation – or disease.

The sympathetic counsellor helps the sick person to accept unpalatable and unresolved truths. Then healing can begin. The next step on the gentle path is to show the patient how to 'make up his mind' to get well again.

The Mental Techniques Which Work

First comes relaxation. This doesn't mean slumping in an armchair to read the newspaper or watch television. There's more to it than that.

At the BCHC relaxation exercises teach the cancer patient to recognise tension in the body, and then create exactly the opposite effect, which is deep physical and mental relaxation.

First of all, participants find a comfortable position. Some people like to sit cross-legged on the floor, others prefer to lie on their backs. Sitting on a straight-backed chair which gives a little support to the spine and is high enough to allow the feet to rest flat on the floor, is another perfectly good position for the relaxation exercises.

The room should be dimly lit, but not dark and well ventilated, but not cold. Remove shoes, loosen tight clothing, close your eyes and you are ready to begin.

Start at the feet and, working your way up through the body, concentrate on each part. First tense and then relax the muscles of the toes, ankles, calves, thighs, buttocks, hips, hands, arms, shoulders and neck; screw up your face, clench your jaw and then let your face go slack. Allow the tongue to sink to the floor of the mouth. Concentrate on the slackness which you have created in every part of your body. Focus your thoughts on what it feels like to be at ease.

To accompany the relaxation exercises, the patient learns to establish a regular pattern of breathing. When we are born, breathing is the first thing we have to learn to do. If we don't, we die. Quite often a baby is brought into the world in adverse circumstances owing to our methods of childbirth. The world seems a hostile place. The infant may not breathe. If he doesn't, he will receive a good whack – so starts life in a state of fear and anger instead of loving tranquillity. Consequently, very fundamental habits are learnt to be connected with breathing so that overcoming wrong breathing and learning to breathe naturally in a relaxed way is of great psychological importance. It is amazing how many psychological problems resolve when right breathing is learned. Discover the rate which is personally comfortable for you. Then, as you breathe in through the nostrils, gently inflate your stomach, perhaps to a silent count of four. Then, slowly exhale, allowing the stomach to flatten, perhaps to the count of six.

With practice it won't be necessary to go through every section of the body first tensing and then relaxing it. All you will need to do is take up your position, regulate your breathing and concentrate on creating a sense of heaviness in your body. This will enable you to slip quite easily into a state of complete ease. It is important to realise that the meditative state is what it is necessary to achieve. It is not the degree of muscular relaxation or the position that it is done in that is important. These are only ways of learning how to carry meditation into ordinary life as a part of it. The Zen Buddhists, the Sufis and the Hindus do this. Of course, it is all called by different names but it is the same thing. The ability to do this in life greatly enhances its quality. One learns to stand outside oneself, observing the reactions of the mind and the body in response to the various events of life and one has a much greater degree of self-control and intensity of living than is otherwise possible. It is a hard life to be at the mercy of one's habits. It should never be forgotten that it is the habits we don't know about that rule us completely, simply because we are not aware of them.

Biofeedback Devices

So often, tensed-up and fearful newcomers to the centre have great difficulty with these relaxation exercises. If modern technology helps to cut corners and achieve results, so much the better. There are several electrical devices which can monitor the depth of relaxation achieved by an individual. This enables the patient to recognise and then generate the feelings which accompany a state of complete relaxation.

One so-called biofeedback device works on the principle of skin resistance. Two small electrodes are held in the hand. An electrical current is passed between them (which the patient doesn't feel) and variations in the moisture content of the palm are registered on a dial. When the subject is tense there is more moisture in the skin than when he is relaxed. Thus, it is possible to watch the meter needle and learn the feelings which cause it to swing towards the reading which indicates a relaxed state.

Another aid to learning the art of relaxation is the Alpha Stimulator which has been used for some time now. A red lamp flickering at the frequency of 4–28 cycles per second, induces corresponding Alpha and Theta Rhythms. The energy levels in someone who is seriously ill, are often pulsing at low levels. The stroboscope then stimulates correct brainwave patterns. Excitable people are soothed by the pulsing light. But once feelings associated with the flow of alpha rhythms are recognised, with practice the patient is then able to generate these without the help of the gadgetry.

Yet another biofeedback system is the EMG. This registers tension in specific muscles, the kind which causes chronic headaches or impedes proper circulation to the extremities. Once the trouble spots have been charted by this kind of electrical monitoring then the patient can concentrate on these problem areas when doing the relaxation exercises.

Similarly, the system called The Mind Mirror is another aid to achieving specific brainwave patterns. Electrodes are taped to the head and patients learn to associate the sensations which correspond to the brainwaves on the monitor and in this way find out how to exercise mental control over muscle tone.

Even without access to biofeedback it is possible to learn deep relaxation merely by the regular practice of breathing exercises and concentrating the mind on 'becoming empty'. But obviously newcomers with no previous experience of these mental therapies do get encouragement from a visible indication of self-achieved inner calm.

The art of learning therapeutic relaxation touches on the exciting realms of metaphysics where essential truths are often concealed in apparent paradox. To explain this, take the example of 'diminishing returns' when the more you try the less you achieve. Everyone has experienced this. For instance, on the spur of the moment you must recall a name. It's on the tip of your tongue but the harder you try to remember the more it evades you. Then sometime later, when nothing could be further from your thoughts, you remember it. The information you needed was there but 'will power' blocked the lines of communication.

So it is with the mind-and-matter healing techniques. Extreme effort is counter-productive. Willpower has little to do with these gentle exercises. Willingness, on the other hand, most certainly does!

The Zen saying 'stop trying and it will do itself' explains the paradox of 'masterful inactivity'. Make a conscious effort to 'let go' and the lines of self-communication are opened up for the healing messages which are built into the Mental Imagery exercises.

Autogenic Training is also called autosuggestion, mental

imagery and self-hypnosis. All these are forms of meditation.

According to physiologists, because the human body is composed of carbon, iron, nitrogen, oxygen, calcium, phosphorous, silicon and so on, we contain the biological ingredients for a perfect electrical battery.

Every living cell carries either a negative or a positive charge. It is the efficient interaction of repulsion and attraction which keeps us going. What we eat, drink and think enables the human power-house to re-charge itself. Top it up with the wrong mixture and there are starting problems.

In health we are literally 'dynamic'. When health is allowed to fail, we become increasingly 'power-less'.

So that energy flow mentioned earlier, is a continual electrical exchange between external surroundings and the biological battery. It's our autonomic nervous system which plugs the internal life force into the external stimulators, bearing in mind that all living particles of matter are electrically charged.

The translation of thought into physiological reactions has already been illustrated by the 'flight or fight' response to fear. We think we are afraid so we start gulping oxygen. Oxygen particles are electrically charged. Extra oxygen in the bloodstream prompts the heart to beat faster and to send tiny impulses to the muscles. The muscles respond by becoming tense. Other electrical impulses switch off the digestive processes and divert blood from skin capillaries to the emergency services in deeper parts of the body, so we become pale with fright. The body has prepared itself for action.

When we think we are safe, our intake of oxygen slows down and all the electrical messengers which alerted the body for action, go into reverse. Then the body relaxes.

All this happens without conscious control. It is reflex action.

In meditation the cancer patient deliberately switches off all external stimuli by regulating the breathing, by putting the body into an unresponsive state.

Brain rhythms slow down from the Beta waves which pulse when the brain is working at normal levels of consciousness (which is awareness) to the slow Alpha rhythms. When Alpha rhythms predominate, the imaginative, intuitive side of our brain is pre-eminent, the side which is usually beyond our conscious control.

When practising meditation at home without the help of biofeedback meters, there are two distinctive signs which will indicate the flow of Alpha rhythms. Either the person will feel a featherweight pressure band across the forehead or experience a sensation of lightness in the body. And when Alpha rhythms start to flow, magical things begin to happen.

The body's need for oxygen decreases, blood pressure drops and in a state which is somewhere between waking and sleeping it becomes possible for the individual to liberate the emotional blockages which have been holding up the healing processes.

This is a somewhat simplistic description of a highly complex system. It leaves out the indefinable ingredient. Call it Soul or Spirit or Super Ego, there is the mysterious plus-factor which is released through meditation.

When the patient is in a meditative state, the therapist will ask him to make a mental picture of how he sees the cancer inside his body. Then how he sees his natural body defences working to overcome it. He is then asked to visualise himself as a fit and healthy person again.

It is important that the mental image is not a negative one where the disease is the powerful aggressor and the body defences the weak opponents. It's the positive mental picture which is going to stimulate your immune system to fight cancer.

One cancer patient pictured her cancer as flurries of snowflakes. Each time she meditated she summoned a flow of warmth and loving to melt them out of existence.

Another saw his disease as the only kind of food enjoyed by shoals of glittering fish which swam through his body gobbling it up.

Someone else imagined his defence system as white knights going into battle. Then, after some months of using this mental image when he meditated, this particular patient told his therapist that for some reason he was finding it impossible to recreate the picture in his mind. All he could see was his white knights riding into battle and then becoming confused and somehow lost. Much to this patient's relief, the therapist had a ready explanation.

There were no more enemy cancer cells for the knights to destroy. Subsequent tests confirmed that this patient was indeed free of cancer.

However you choose to visualise your cancer and the way your immune system is working to overcome it, always select a picture which depicts the good and strong defence system overcoming the weak and confused cancer cells.

Cancer is not something which has come from outside your body, like a virus or bacterial infection which the immune system recognises as alien matter and mobilises against. Cancer is a part of your essential self, formed by cells which once functioned for the health and growth of the whole system before they 'forgot' their purpose and began growing in a hostile fashion. Even so, your cancer is still made of the same substances which form the rest of your body, so don't choose a symbolic image which involves too much violence.

Cancer takes a long time to get established and produce the symptoms which first made you aware of it. Gentle therapy measures also need time and persistence on your part, before they become effective.

The advantages of relaxation and visualisation techniques are soon apparent.

1 These exercises reduce fear. Fear comes from feelings of helplessness, of being unable to control the course of disease. Visualisation exercises enable you to regain control of the situation.
2 These exercises really help to prepare the way for the important changes which need to be made both

internally and externally when you follow the gentle path to recovery.

3 Visualisation influences the overall efficiency of your immune system which is not selective. Stimulating it to combat cancer means that if you happen to be suffering from other ailments, self-healing will also have a beneficial effect on these.

4 Superficially meditation will not change the kind of person you are, but it will enable you to view your illness and your way of living in an entirely new and constructive way. Meditation builds up your self-confidence.

Pathways of the Mind

Through meditation it is possible to reverse the disease process by using the same neurological pathways which made it possible in the first place. But it is regular practice of all the wholistic therapies which provides the key to restoring whole health.

Basically these are self-help methods but it is to be hoped that the patient will have the understanding and co-operation of close family members.

Serious Illness is a Family Matter

When someone has reached a state of despair, family support is essential. Although the friendliness and compassion of the Bristol therapists is second to none and many of them have already been through the 'dark valley' themselves, in the end they can't be expected to provide a limitless rescue service for the cancer patient.

Ultimately, the patient must go home and make the necessary life-giving adjustments within his or her own family circle.

Of course it's important that the patient's family help to

prepare the diet and make sure that quiet times are set aside for meditation. But understanding how the patient really feels is even more important. As with any life-threatening illness, the patient may have wild swings of mood: emotions of fear, anger, self-pity, guilt and many others. All place an undue strain on family life unless the rest of the household understand how to cope with them.

The patient's family may well have their guilt feelings too, for being so healthy when the other person is so ill. They may compensate for this by being overprotective and then find this irritates the patient. So the family moves too far the other way and the patient reacts by feeling rejected.

This is when a trained counsellor can offer the kind of advice which enables the family to provide the sick person with a dimension of emotional and practical support which finds a way round these problems.

Nobody who has cancer should ever be made to feel that he can't talk openly about his illness in case others find it upsetting. He may believe he's a 'nuisance' or 'unloved'. Then the family should be prepared to sit down and listen to whatever he has to say and give appropriate and honest reassurance. The family also needs to be allowed to express its anxieties and not hide behind a façade of false optimism. In these circumstances holding back feelings isn't courageous. Courage is finding ways to give free expression to everyone's feelings and not being afraid to show one another all the fears and weaknesses which go with this degree of honesty.

Empty out your emotional pockets, examine what you find, discard the rubbish and put back the valuables. Maybe this kind of emotional springcleaning is long overdue, but everyone concerned will appreciate the relief which follows it.

It is never easy to watch someone you love struggling for life, especially with therapies which may seem so strange. At such a time the sick person needs all the encouragement possible, and only when the family understands all the emotions involved can it best provide this. Then it is possible

to establish a sense of family unity which is second to none
Cancer becomes a learning and growing experience even i
the ultimate healing doesn't happen at a physical level.

Healing

Anyone who has been treated as a 'case' in a busy hospita
or spent an hour waiting for a consultation with their GP
may have sensed that this brand of health *care* is dispensec
without much emphasis on the second word.

At the Bristol Cancer Help Centre, hospitality comes first.
This in itself sets the scene for healing. Under one roof are
gathered those able to minister to the sick person's needs a
all levels of being – physical, spiritual and emotional.

Once this was a fundamental ethic in the practice o
medicine. 'Hospital', 'hospice' and 'hospitality' were one
and the same. Nowadays, it is only in the hospices for
terminal care that true hospitality exists. In our moderr
society, the ethic of wholistic medicine is reserved for the
dying.

Healing demands little of the patient. It neither imposes
nor presupposes any particular religious faith. The patient's
trust and 'willingness to be healed' reinforces the effect but
if these are lacking, healing will still take place.

Either by physical contact (the laying on of hands) or by
the transmission of healing thoughts, the healer creates a
channel of energy between himself and the sick person.
Exactly what or where this energy comes from is not clear,
although the technique known as Kirlian Photography has
captured the remarkable increase in the energy field which
surrounds the hands of a healer in action. The Mind
Mirror, which gives a simultaneous two-sided read-out o
the brain waves, shows that, when healing, healers have
symmetrical Alpha and Theta wave patterns which are not
found in non-healers. Healers are capable of inducing the
same pattern in the brains of those they are healing.

The popular concept of healing as a 'miracle cure' is a sensational one. This sometimes happens, but as already intimated, healing occurs on more than just the physical level. Spectacular relief from a serious ailment has followed a healing session, but more frequently, healing creates the inner easiness' which unblocks the patient's unconscious resistance to the possibility of getting well again.

Sometimes the ministrations of a healer are only effective at a nonphysical level when the sick person is helped to make the ultimate change – which is the transition from life to death. Then healing is one of the gentle therapies which dissolves the pain and fear which might otherwise degrade this event.

Barbara: A Personal Story

Shortly after hearing a BBC radio documentary I made about my experience of gentle therapies, I got a telephone call from a woman called Barbara. As she lived in the next town, I offered to visit her.

Barbara was in her early 40s, a lecturer in chemistry at the local polytechnic and a highly qualified and intelligent woman.

She had begun life in Canada, the only child of Jewish parents who had fled from Germany during the Nazi persecutions. These parents centred their love and attention on Barbara, encouraging her to do well at her studies. In due course Barbara fulfilled their expectations. When they died, Barbara applied for a teaching post at an English college and made her home here.

I went to see Barbara several times between Spring and the end of the year. As we became better acquainted I recognised much of myself in her, before I started on the gentle path therapies.

Barbara was not the kind of person to suffer fools gladly. She was very much an 'all-or-nothing' type of person, expecting high standards of herself and the same from those around her. This limited her ability to make close friendships. But although she gave the impression of being a strong, self-sufficient person, underneath there was someone entirely different. As she told me, she longed to give and receive deep affection but always held back. Exposing her soft centre, she believed, would make her too vulnerable to the kind of emotional hurts which she might not be able to handle.

Five years before I met Barbara she'd been operated on for breast cancer and had remained well; until the married man with whom she was having an affair, ended it. Within a few months Barbara's health started to deteriorate.

She listened with a slightly cynical smile whenever I described the vitamin therapies and diet which might help her. To her credit, she made a thorough study of the subject before declaring that in her opinion such 'unscientific' methods lacked credibility. However, she was interested in the visualisation techniques which did not conflict with her orthodox training.

'What I want is someone who can help me find a reason for all this,' she used to say.

Eventually, Barbara was admitted to the local hospice for terminal nursing. Staffed by exceptionally sensitive people, here at last love and care was lavished on her, a woman who, despite her intellectual achievements, had never managed to attract the one thing in life she wanted above all else: unconditional love.

In the hospice she was surrounded by people ready to sit down and listen to what she had to say about herself, about her illness, about her dying.

Shortly after Barbara died, the medical director of the hospice wrote me this letter: '… I am returning the books and literature you lent to Barbara. I have read some of these but am afraid I remain unconvinced of the value of Laetrile.

'… during her stay with us Barbara felt that although we did not have as positive an approach to her illness as she would have liked, she found the staff very supportive. Her death was extremely peaceful. She slept for the last 48 hours.

'... whilst with us, Barbara used to say: "It's life I'm afraid of, not death." '

What Does the Sick Person Need?

At Bristol the counsellor is always sensitive to the patient's needs. Not all patients actually wish to get well again, so it is important that the therapist acknowledges this withdrawal, and respects it.

There is also the person who despite a genuine attempt to fight for recovery, does not respond to the gentle therapies, usually when the disease is already far advanced and more aggressive forms of treatment have caused irremedial damage. Then at a purely physical level the system can't repair itself. But here again, gentle therapies, lovingly applied, enrich the quality of the life that remains.

Lifelines

Whilst explaining the wholistic therapies, I've tried to be factual. Nobody should get the impression that these are quick and easy ways to regain health because in most cases they are not. What they can be is a lifeline which you can use to haul yourself back to safety. Then, so often, the sick person comes through the experience to enjoy an entirely fresh and invigorating view of life and living.

The gentle therapy path needs courage, perseverance and the ability to regard what you are doing to help yourself with a sense of adventure. But it can be a lonely trail.

Since this book first appeared, Cancer Help Support Groups have sprung up all over the British Isles.* Most of these seek to perpetuate the wholistic programme as pioneered at Bristol. They provide a regular meeting place for cancer patients and their families so they can get together and feel that they are not alone in the struggle to regain their health by self-healing methods.

It is now four years since the Gentle Way therapies first appeared in the UK, and there are now a growing number of patients who are able to testify to the benefit they have derived from them. And many of these are able to depend upon their doctors for support and encouragement.

* Further information about Support Groups can be obtained from the Association for New Approaches to Cancer (address p.175).

10   THE GENTLE WAY AHEAD

In July 1983 the new residential Bristol Cancer Help Centre was officially opened by HRH The Prince of Wales. In his speech he said:

'... The great value, it seems to me, of the type of treatment provided here is not that extravagant claims are made on its behalf, but that it does no positive harm to the patient ... for so much depends on marshalling the psychological and spiritual forces of the patient to tackle the appalling afflictions which have arisen. But marshalling these resources, together with the remarkable ones belonging to Mother Nature, are not carried out in direct competition with what could be termed as "the orthodox approach" to treating the patient, but in a complementary sense.

'From my own personal point of view, I think it is only right that a patient should be free to try a different form of treatment if he or she feels that little progress is being made in, for instance, what may be referred to as a drug-based form of treatment ...'

Since the original Centre first opened in 1980, a steady stream of patients has gone to Bristol to find out more about wholistic therapies. Only 30 per cent decided to use them. The remainder felt the effort and changes involved were more than they could manage on their own. But out of that 30 per cent, in every case the quality of life was improved and many patients, after being told by their orthodox consultants that there was 'nothing more to be done', managed to stabilise the course of their disease.

But despite this, and the willingness of patients to testify in public that they have successfully used the therapies, in the main the medical profession still refuses to acknowledge the validity of 'unscientific' treatments based on the nutritional approach.

Yet in 1957 the World Health Organisation was cautioning western nations about the long-term dangers of artificial methods of food production as people's eating habits changed from natural foodstuffs to highly processed ones. WHO predicted a large increase in chronic ailments such as arthritis, heart disease and cancer, but in the immediate post-war years governments preoccupied with economic recovery were not pausing to consider the far-off future.

As for the people, after ten years of a National Health Service which promised to take care of every man, woman and child 'from the womb to the tomb', they were already convinced that responsibility for their health care was safely in the hands of the medical establishment.

Now the future is here. More than thirty years of chemicalised farming, foods de-natured by processing and other forms of environmental pollution have exacted a heavy price in the number of people suffering from chronic degenerative diseases such as cancer. The incidence increases year by year and affects not just the old. The grim statistic that one-in-four people can expect to get cancer is spread across the entire age-range.

The medical establishment's response to ecological mayhem has been – and still is – to pour millions into researching drug treatments, many of which have added to patient problems in the form of iatrogenic (drug-induced) diseases.

The overall annual health-care bill in the UK is around £16 billion and rising. In 1983, out of this total, £2000 million was spent on drug treatments. The money spent annually on health education and preventive measures is currently less than 10 per cent and dropping. And wherever vested interests are involved, even this expenditure amounts to little more than a token gesture.

Take, for instance, this vexed question of health and the tobacco industry.

Tobacco

The link between smoking and cancer has been proved beyond dispute, but the ban on advertising and the health warnings on cigarette packets hasn't made any difference to the smoking habits of the nation.

In the UK, £150 million is spent annually on hospital care for people with tobacco-related complaints such as heart disease, bronchitis, lung and bladder cancer. Prescriptions issued by GPs for home treatment for these problems account for another £80-90 million. But this expenditure is a drop in the ocean compared with government revenue from the sale of tobacco.

In any one year this amounts to more than £4000 million. And what use is the embargo on TV advertising for cigarettes if TV companies are allowed to screen major sports events sponsored by tobacco companies?

Obviously when it comes to smoking the individual is free to make choices. In other areas of community health, this is not always possible. And for every identified public health hazard – such as smoking – there are equally dangerous hidden risks which the general public has little chance of avoiding.

Fluoridation

In the UK at this moment, health authorities are imposing fluoridation of water supplies when every other European country has banned the use of a substance which has been shown to be a slow-acting poison.

Tooth decay has been a serious problem for western civilisation since just after the last war when the end of food rationing heralded the birth of the food processing industry. The national diet soon became loaded with refined carbohydrates.

In the early 1940s a US dental researcher investigating

the cause of the exceptionally good teeth in people living in a certain part of Texas, discovered that their water contained a rather high concentration of fluoride. He assumed (erroneously as we now know) that it was fluoride in the water which prevented tooth decay.

It also happened that about this time the aluminium industry was looking for ways to dispose of the waste product occasioned by their manufacturing processes. This was fluoride. By a happy coincidence, improved dental health could go hand-in-hand with improved profits for this industry.

Forty years after putting fluoride into water supplies in order to prevent dental decay, it has proved to be a mistake.

Surveys confirm that children fed on a proper diet which is low in refined carbohydrates, grow up with perfectly good teeth. Secondly, a whole mass of studies made both in the United States and in this country show that not only is cancer linked to fluoride but so are a number of other distressing ailments.

In 1977 the International Society for Fluoride Research at the Oxford Union stated that new and conclusive data clearly established that artificially fluoridated water can be strikingly harmful to some humans. After checking and rechecking a study of some 20m people in the USA, it was reported that increased cancer death rates commenced within a few years after the initiation of fluoridation, with marked, continued increases thereafter, and that from the age of 45, one in ten cancer deaths was due to fluoridated public water supply. (Yiamouyiannis, *Fluoridation and Cancer*, 1977.)

Evidence which challenged the National Cancer Institute's insistence that 'fluoride is harmless' (which is the view taken by most UK physicians) was given by researchers from Japan, Holland, Denmark, Germany and Greece.

'Fluoride can be linked with mongolism and cancer,' said the Oxford scientists. 'At a time when the whole of Europe has rejected fluoride because they are afraid of hitherto unrecognised systemic abnormalities which may arise through a lifetime's consumption of this enzyme inhibitor and poison, Britain is pushing ahead with fluoridation.'

At best, fluoridation will only delay the onset of tooth decay in children by, on average, one tooth for one year. As shown in the US studies, it will increase substantially the deaths from cancer of the parents and grandparents of the children whose teeth it is supposed to benefit.

Misinformed politicians and health authorities zealously expose a large proportion of the public to the risk of side-effects from mass medication designed to protect children from tooth decay. Responsible parents who provide a healthy diet for the family, can do this at home. Or, if they wish, they can get the dentist to paint fluoride onto the child's teeth.

Forty per cent of the American population have fluoride in their drinking water. So far in the UK it is only ten per cent but if a persistent and ill-informed lobby of health authorities isn't stopped, they will go ahead with plans to increase this percentage.

Nobody can say to what extent the prevalence of cancer today is a legacy from past environmental abuse. But slowly the truth is filtering through.

The Hidden Enemy: Radiation

An article in the October 24 issue of the British Medical Association's prestigious journal *The Lancet* and written by T. Alan Phillips, revealed that the incidence of leukemia in Britain in 1957 was five times higher than in 1920, a staggering increase. The suggestion that this was the result of radioactivity released into the atmosphere years before, is not such a wild supposition as it would appear.

Between 1945 and 1963 not only were there the Hiroshima and Nagasaki detonations but also nuclear bomb testing by all major nations.

Governments of the day constantly assured people that there was little, if any, danger from radioactive fall-out.

The US Department of Defence alone conducted 235 'announced' atmospheric nuclear weapon tests between 1945 and the Nuclear Test Ban Treaty in 1963. During the course of these, 250,000 American soldiers were deliberately exposed to ionizing radiation at the Nevada test-sites and on various Pacific islands such as Bikini Atoll, in order to 'observe their reactions'. All the men were told that 'radiation was harmless' and consequently no protective clothing was issued.

In July 1982 a report from the National Association of Atomic Veterans published the results of a medical follow-up on 700 veterans from these tests. The report makes horrific reading, not only because of what has happened to the ex-soldiers, but to their children also.

A quarter of the veterans have developed leukemia or other cancerous conditions and the following figures relate to the 345 children born to this group: 44 miscarriages; 23 stillbirths and early deaths; 192 births with serious congenital defects.

Abnormalities in these children ranged from mental retardation to sterility but mostly concerned the appearance of cancer tumours. Some children had multiple disabilities.

After the notorious Windscale nuclear reactor accident in 1957, the incidence of leukemia in the area rose in the next few years to 36 times the national average. The complete cost in terms of genetic damage has yet to be assessed.

Disposal of waste products from nuclear power stations is yet another problem which, if we let it, will create a legacy of trouble for our children's children.

Radioactive caesium discharged into the Irish Sea has already built up a radioactive sediment on the seabed and the Ministry of Agriculture and Fisheries confirm that radioactive material from Windscale has moved into the North Sea.

Plutonium waste released into the English Channel from the French nuclear reprocessing plant at The Hague has already contaminated the northern coastline of Germany. (Nicholas Hildyard, *Cover Up*, 1980.)

When it comes to radioactive elements, we are dealing with a whole new scientific entity. What has happened in the past is undoubtedly partly responsible for the rising incidence of cancer.

Freedom to Choose

Cancer is a tragic illness. The average person doesn't understand the nature of this disease and believes the allopathic specialists are prescribing the only treatments for it. The so-called 'experts', having invested their reputations in cancer drugs and machinery, have a monopoly on cancer care. They are unlikely to relinquish this in favour of treatments which include carrot juice, beansprouts, and meditation!

As one doctor put it, when told by a cancer patient that she intended going on a special cleansing diet:

'Surely you don't think *rabbit food* can cure cancer!' This facetious remark was a graphic example of the medical profession's defensive response to (1) the cancer patient's attempt to take some responsibility for his or her own treatments and (2) any challenge to their authority and expertise.

Yet as Brian Inglis quotes in his book *The Diseases of Civilisation*: 'Lay people should understand that there are no real experts in research on cancer or on any of the other diseases to which they have no answers. The failure of cancer research to achieve substantial results and its failure to demonstrate why and how cancer develops, indicate that the so-called experts are *failed* experts.'

Fortunately there are many people alive today because they refused to allow the 'experts' to have the last word.

Going it Alone

Four years ago Eunice Durban, a widow in her late 60s living in Chester, was told that she only had six weeks to live when a recurring breast cancer spread out of control.

After undergoing mastectomy for the primary tumour in 1975, Mrs Durban remained well for the next four years. Then one morning, she slipped whilst collecting the milk off her doorstep and bruised her chest. Despite radiotherapy treatment, in a few weeks her body had bloated from ten stones to 15 stones and she was told that there was nothing more that could be done to help her.

At this point, Mrs Durban's daughter, Eileen, took her to a naturopath doctor. They returned home determined to try the Gerson nutritional therapy programme.

As her mother was far too ill to prepare the fresh-pressed vegetables and fruit juices she needed to drink every hour of her waking day, or to give herself frequent coffee enemas to stimulate detoxification, Eileen undertook the tasks. But there were practical difficulties.

In a suburban area, obtaining organically grown vegetables for the juices was almost impossible. Then there were the financial problems such as the cost of an expensive electrical juicer and the necessary vitamin injections and supplements.

Mrs Durban found she was spending most of her retirement pension each week on these life-giving necessities. For the programme did save her life.

When I telephoned Mrs Durban in December 1982, she was leading a near-normal life again and continuing a modified form of the Gerson diet which continues to cost her about £20 a week. But if the story of Eunice Durban is remarkable, the effect that Gerson therapy had on her daughter Eileen is even more astonishing.

Since childhood Eileen had suffered from epilepsy which subjected her to three or four fits in a single day. When she began helping her mother with the diet, Eileen decided she'd try it too. That was three years ago. Today Eileen

Gough has no further signs of epilepsy.

Orthodox medical opinion would say that either the original diagnosis on Mrs Durban was at fault (in which case why did she need a mastectomy?) or that the radiotherapy treatment produced a delayed effect.

As for the cure Eileen managed to achieve by nutritional methods when extensive (and expensive) drug treatments failed, this has elicited no comment.

Gerson Got it Right

Another woman struggling alone to cure herself of cancer was Mrs Rosemary Hazell of Bishop's Stortford in Hertfordshire.

Before her illness, Rosemary worked as a clinical psychologist. In 1977 she was diagnosed as having skin cancer (melanoma), a condition which is usually regarded as incurable by conventional treatments.

The first time I phoned Rosemary for this book, she asked me to call back in an hour as she was about to have a coffee enema. When next we spoke, she explained that she'd been on the strict Gerson regime for a year and was finding it extremely hard to manage on her own.

Initially her husband was able to help out, but only reluctantly. Eventually the marriage broke up.

'So many men can't cope with adversity,' Rosemary said. 'My husband was very angry because I was trying to cure myself. He felt I should rely on my consultants.'

Not only was the marital separation an emotional shock for Rosemary Hazell, but it also left her living on social security. Fortunately, a financial sponsor scheme originating from the Gerson Clinic in Mexico for patients experiencing financial hardship enabled her to continue the therapy.

Fresh vegetables, fruit, liver injections, and fresh coffee for the enemas, cost Rosemary Hazell between £100 and £200 a month. Although her GP helped with injections and generally gave his moral support, he was unable to prescribe any of the dietary items Rosemary needed because they are not drugs.

A distributor of organically-grown vegetables in London supplied Rosemary with her weekly requirements of fruit and vegetables, and the two pounds of fresh liver which features on the Gerson diet was obtained from farmers who reared calves by traditional farming methods.

When she was not at school, Rosemary's eight-year-old daughter Rowena helped prepare the hourly juices.

'Rowena says when she grows up she's going to teach other children about the Gerson diet,' Rosemary told me. 'She wants everybody to know how juices made me come alive again.'

In the summer of 1984, Rosemary Hazell was back at work in her hospital department, all signs of her melanoma gone.

The medical establishment ignores the value of what Eunice Durban and Rosemary Hazell have achieved by their own determined efforts. Yet to quote the stories of just two women who have used biological medicine to overcome their cancers is to overlook the scores of other people (mostly in the USA) who have put up a similar fight and won through.

The Californian housewife Jaquie Davison wrote a book called *Cancer Winner; How I purged myself of Melanoma* which describes how Gerson therapy restored her to health. The Cancer Control Society in Los Angeles publishes long lists of people who have also fought cancer with gentle therapies.

It seems inconceivable that in the face of this over-whelming evidence the orthodox medical profession can afford to dismiss naturopathic treatments for cancer as 'unscientific' and 'unproven'.

Health for the New Age

Eradicating the fear of cancer by educating people as to the origins of this illness is the prime objective of every group and organisation working in the field of non-toxic cancer therapy. First and foremost is the Cancer Control Society of Los Angeles.

For more than a decade this Society has been prominent in its efforts to inform and educate the public about reputable non-toxic cancer therapies and reliable practitioners. It has vigorously campaigned against medical authorities that deny cancer patients the right to have the treatments of their choice.

'Knowledge,' says Betty Lee Morales, nutritionist president of the CCS, 'is your greatest weapon. Public opinion is the greatest force. When you know how to protect yourself against cancer and then choose not to, that is your personal decision. If you do know and accept the nutritional truths and wish to apply them, but are prevented from doing so by your own government, that is tyranny.'

For some years now the WHO has been trying to encourage member states to incorporate traditional medicine into their health systems. In the UK osteopathy, healing and acupuncture are now officially regarded as 'respectable' by the medical profession. As a result, an increasing number of informed patients are turning to so-called 'alternative' practitioners for help with complaints which their allopathic doctors seem unable to treat.

In 1982 the Threshold Foundation of Cambridge published a directory of nearly 8000 practitioners of complementary therapies in the UK. The very fact that these people exist demonstrates public discontent with the current model of health care determined to treat diseases not people. The success of a series of London conferences on gentle therapy measures for the treatment of cancer seemed to confirm that at long last people are prepared to question the validity of orthodox cancer care.

In November 1979 the first of three seminars was held at the Royal Society of Medicine in London, under the auspices of 'Health for the New Age'. Over the following three years, leading proponents of gentle therapy cancer treatments, who were also trained in allopathic medicine, were invited to speak.

Dr Hans Neiper, the highly-respected German cancer specialist who combines orthodox treatments with non-toxic programmes, was one such lecturer.

Dr Neiper showed the audience X-rays of patients with widespread bone cancer before having his treatment and then some months later when the X-rays showed healed bone tissue. Neiper's method includes Laetrile and food factor supplements together with conventional medicine.

Dr Ernesto Contreras was another conference speaker who talked about the methods he has been using at his Mexican-based Del Mar Clinic, a wholistic programme similar to the one developed at Bristol.

Both these doctors have been closely involved with non-toxic cancer care for *more than twenty years*. They had on record thousands of cancer cases and from these were able to state that even in terminal cases, gentle methods had prolonged life with increased quality. Fifteen per cent of their 'hopeless' cases had recovered to lead normal lives.

In orthodox cancer treatment spontaneous remissions are a rarity.

Carl and Stephanie Simonton were also invited to speak at the 'New Approaches to Cancer' conferences, describing their work with mental imagery techniques which has now become 'required reading' for students of psychology at the University of California at Berkeley.

From Holland came representatives of the Moerman Clinic and Dr Hans Moolenburgh who, in his home-town of Haarlem, has for many years been giving cancer patients Laetrile in conjunction with a strict dietary programme.

Then in March 1983 the BBC Television series *A Gentle Way With Cancer* gave millions of viewers the opportunity to follow the progress of six patients at the Bristol Cancer Help Centre as they tried to control the course of their disease.

The London-based conferences, many more television and radio documentaries and discussion programmes, together with outspoken articles in the press, are gradually removing the mystique and fear surrounding the once-taboo subject of cancer.

People are talking more about the disease, and learning more about its biological origins and the natural self-help methods which can lead to recovery from it.

There is still a long way to go before we can reverse and re-dress the damage done to both our external and internal environments.

In her book *Silent Spring*, Rachel Carson wrote: 'The balance of nature is ... in a constant state of adjustment. Man too is a part of this balance. Sometimes the balance is in his favour, sometimes – and all too often through his own activities – it is shifted to his disadvantage.'

The last thirty years of medicinal drugs and artificial farming methods have denied the individual the opportunity to enjoy an uncontaminated environment.

Wind, rain, rivers, seas, and seepage spread the poisons. Governments do not publicise the plain facts and the man-in-the-street, intent upon the orchestration of his external needs, forgets that his internal rhythms dance to a more primitive tune.

Whose Health is it Anyway?

The human body is equipped with the most intricate self-healing system – if only we learn how to allow it to operate unhindered.

When we violate the elementary laws of health or subject the body to severe stresses or other adverse environmental factors, it reacts with one or more acute symptoms. This may be pain or fever, bowel upsets, high blood pressure or indigestion – but whatever the distress signals, these only mean that the healthy body is taking defensive action against whatever has harmed its natural equilibrium. In our ignorance, we often misinterpret these acute symptoms and call them illnesses or disease.

Instead of resting and fasting to assist natural healing mechanisms, we hurry for medical help and 'instant' drug remedies. In this way a vicious circle is established.

Impeded by unnatural medicaments, self-healing mechanisms begin to function less efficiently, and since the cause of the disequilibrium remains, the symptoms return. More medicines further reduce the efficiency of the immune system, and so the internal stage is set for chronic illnesses.

The rapid development of the chemical and physical sciences in the last two centuries has had a most negative influence upon medical thinking and slowed down the progress of the true healing arts.

In his book *How To Get Well*, the naturopath doctor Paavo Airola writes:

'Unbelievable as it may seem, the twentieth-century concept of disease is not much different from the primitive voodoo concept. The only difference is that the "evil spirits" have been replaced by "evil germs". We believe that disease "strikes" the unsuspecting, and the job of the modern medicine man is to kill or drive out the evil intruders with magic power from medicine bottle or injection needle.

'Disease is not a negative condition which should be combatted and suppressed. It is a positive, constructive process initiated by the body in an attempt to restore health.'

Biological medicine is based on the premise that all illnesses have the same basic underlying causes. They are biochemical and metabolic disorders brought about by prolonged physical and mental stresses which have not been properly recognised by the patient.

Therefore the only effective way to cure the 'disease' is to eliminate the causes, as far as possible with methods which do not interfere or damage the natural healing properties of the body.

With special dietary factors, cleansing programmes, specific vitamins, juices, herbs, and other natural substances, the symptoms (diseases) will disappear – not because the therapist has cured them, but because *there is no more reason for their existence.*

Self-healing has been given the *only* assistance it requires to restore the system to well-being.

Cancer is a disease of civilisation. It is the end result of health-destroying living and eating habits, and the abundance of carcinogens in today's food, water and air.

It is to be hoped that before long the naturopathic view of health will influence the current mechanistic medical model. Then at last the value of mobilising the patient's own life force to turn 'dis-ease' into 'ease' will become self-evident.

Whole health is a heritage which belongs to everyone. Eventually it is biological medicine which will safeguard that heritage. Then perhaps we can really begin to reverse the tides of chronic disease and look forward to a world without cancer.

GLOSSARY OF TERMS

Allopathic Treatment with drugs

Amino acids Simple chemical substances contained in protein. There are nine essential amino acids which are not all found in poor diets

Anorexia Loss of appetite

Anti-oxidant Any substance which protects against decomposition

Bioflavinoids Natural substance in Vitamin C which assists absorption

Biopsy Tissue fragment taken for analysis

Carcinogens Substances (usually in the environment) which produce cancer *eg*. asbestos dust, nitrates, etc.

Chemotherapy Treatment of cancer with poisonous drugs

Chromosome Within one chromosome is a large collection of genes; each gene determines one element of hereditary make-up

Collagen A protein component of all connective tissue. Many processes of ageing (*eg*. wrinkles) are due to derangement of collagen

Cytotoxics Chemical drugs which poison cancer cells used in chemotherapy.

DNA Acronym for deoxyribonucleic acid; the component of a cell which governs reproduction

Dysplastic Cell changes

Empirical Results based on observations not theory

Enzymes Biochemical compounds which orchestrate the organisation and arrangement of living matter without changing themselves. They are catalysts and exert their own electrical fields

Epithelium Coating or lining tissues *eg*. skin or mucous membrane

Fetor Bad odour from open wounds

Frozen section A tissue specimen is freeze dried until it is hard enough to take a microscopic slice for analysis

Gamma globulin Blood proteins formed in the lymphatic system to protect against specific infections. Part of the immune system

In situ Only in one place

Leukocytes White blood cell

Liver Largest gland in the body. It lies under the diaphragm. It is the principal organ of digestion and excretion

Lymph glands (Lymphatics) Clusters of bean-like structures in various parts of the body. They prevent infection spreading, so form an essential part of the immune system

Mastectomy Surgical removal of breast

Metastases Spread of cancer from primary site to other parts of the body

Mutation Change in structure of the gene which carries the chemical blue-print for correct cell reproduction

Oncologist A tumour specialist

Palliative Treatment which eases symptoms (*eg.* pain) and does nothing to the disease

Pancreas The soft digestive gland which lies behind the stomach and under the liver

Peristalsis Rhythmic contractions of intestines to expel faeces

Prophylactic Preventive treatment

Prostaglandins Hormones which control the production of T-lymphocytes

Remission A temporary dying down of a disease or its symptoms

T-lymphocytes Scavenger blood cells

USEFUL ADDRESSES

The Association for New
Approaches to Cancer
The Seekers Trust
The Close
Addington Park
Nr. Maidstone
Kent ME19 5BL
(Tel: 0732 848336)

British Holistic Medical Assoc.
179 Gloucester Place
London NW1 6DX

The Cancer Control Society
2043 No. Berendo Street
Los Angeles,
Calif. 90027

Natural Therapists

The British Naturopathic and
Osteopathic Association
6 Netherall Gardens
London NW3 5RR
(Tel: 01-435 7830)

The British Homoeopathic
Association
27a Devonshire Street
London W1N 1RJ

The Society of Homoeopaths
59 Norfolk House
Streatham
London SW16

The National Institute of
Medical Herbalists
65 Frant Road
Tunbridge Wells
Kent TH2 5LH

The Faculty of Herbal
Medicine
93 East Avenue
Bournemouth
Hampshire BA3 7BK

The Bristol Cancer Help
Centre
Grove House
Cornwallis Grove
Clifton
Bristol BS8 4PG
(Tel: 0272 743216)
NB: Please enclose SAE for
reply

Healers

The National Federation of
Spiritual Healers
Old Manor Farm Studio
Church Street
Sunbury-on-Thames
Middlesex TW16 6RG
(Tel: 09327 83164)

Spiritualist Association of
Great Britain
33 Belgrave Square,
London SW1

Organic Growers

Henry Doubleday Research
Association
Convent Lane
Bocking
Braintree
Essex CM7 6RW
(Tel: 0376 24083)

The Soil Association
Walnut Tree Manor
Haughley
Stowmarket
Suffolk

Organic Growers Association
Aeron Park
Llangeitho
Dyfed, Wales

Food Watch
High Acre
East Stour
Gillingham
Dorset SP8 5JR

Water Filters

Brighter UK Ltd
51 Ashley Road
Walton-on-Thames
Surrey

Daltons
Slough
Bucks
(Tel: 050 782 655)

SUGGESTED READING

Getting Well Again by Dr Carl and Stephanie Simonton, Bantam Books, paperback

An End to Cancer by Leon Chaitow, Thorsons of Wellingborough

You Can Fight For Your Life by Lawrence LeShan, Evan & Co. Inc., New York, USA

Gerson Therapy: *A Cancer Therapy: Results of Fifty Cases* from Margaret Straus, 97 Bedford Court Mansions, London WC1

World Without Cancer by G. Edward Griffin, Thorsons of Wellingborough

Cancer: How to Prevent It and How to Help Your Doctor Fight It by George E. Berkley Ph.D, Prentice Hall Inc., Englewood Cliffs, New Jersey 07632 USA

A Manual of Self-Healing by E.H. Shattock, Turnstone Press, Wellingborough, North Hants

Cancer and its Nutritional Therapies by R.A. Passwater, Keats Publishing Inc., New Canaan, Conn., USA

The Holistic Approach to Cancer by Ian C.B. Pearce, obtainable from the Association for New Approaches to Cancer

New Hope and Improved Treatments for Cancer Patients by David Holmes, John Wiley

INDEX